The
Gift *of*
Life

The
Gift of
Life

The Reality Behind
Donor Organ Retrieval

Traci Graf, RN

FIREFLY BOOKS

A FIREFLY BOOK

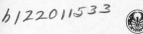

Published by Firefly Books Ltd. 2014
Copyright © 2014 Firefly Books Ltd.
Text Copyright © 2014 Traci Graf
First Printing

Publisher Cataloging-in-Publication Data (U.S.)
A CIP record for this title is available from the Library of Congress.

Library and Archives Canada Cataloguing in Publication
A CIP record for this title is available from Library and Archives Canada.

Published in the United States by
Firefly Books (U.S.) Inc.
P.O. Box 1338, Ellicott Station
Buffalo, New York 14205

Published in Canada by
Firefly Books Ltd.
50 Staples Avenue, Unit 1
Richmond Hill, Ontario L4B 0A7

Cover and interior design: Hartley Millson
Author photo: Jennifer Jacono
Cover photo: uchar/E+/Getty Images
Illustrations: Shutterstock © Hein Nouwens

Printed in Canada

*The publisher gratefully acknowledges the financial support for our publishing
program by the Government of Canada through the Canada Book Fund as
administered by the Department of Canadian Heritage.*

To all transplant coordinators and donor families.

Contents

Introduction

ORGAN TRANSPLANTS ARE A VERY CONTROVERSIAL AND UNIQUE AREA OF medicine. During the time I worked as a Transplant Coordinator (TC), I often noticed that TC's were referred to by hospital staff as "organ vultures" behind our backs. I felt this reference to extremely ugly birds was unfair and short sighted. I did say once in a while to a difficult staff person, "If your kid needed a transplant wouldn't you hope that someone was out there being as ethically aggressive about finding an organ as they could?" That usually shut them up quickly.

Every area of the country has a federally designated Organ Procurement Organization (OPO) that covers the hospitals in their region. I worked in one of the largest regions and an area that had one of the most successful OPO's in the world. We had over 150 hospitals in our region and about 35 TC's to cover them. Each day between six to eight strategically placed TC's were on call somewhere in our large area. I lived right between the rural areas and the big city hospitals, which made me a good option to send either way.

We were a good mix of Registered Nurses (RN's) with various backgrounds and paramedics. I had an unusual background for this job. I started in the Operating Room (OR) when I was 19 years old as a surgical technologist handing instruments to surgeons in many different specialties. I spent 16 years in the OR and learned something from everyone I encountered. In my early 30s I decided to pursue Pathology at medical school, an area of medicine I always found fascinating, diagnosing surgical specimens and autopsies within the hospital setting. I was fortunate enough to have a wonderful group of surgeons, nurses and pathologists mentor me for almost three years, teaching me more than I ever thought was possible. I was about 32, had an 8-month-old daughter, a 6-year-old daughter and an 11-year-old son at home. I was working full time in the OR, taking calls in the OR at night and weekends and taking classes online and on campus at night for premed prerequisites. I worked very hard at trying to get accepted into medical school but it just wasn't what I was meant to do or I wouldn't be writing this book. I switched to nursing school and breezed through most of it because of the background I had and my inquisitive nature. Ironically, I wrote an essay as part of the admissions process for nursing school describing how TC's were my inspiration to become a nurse. In this essay I detailed how the TC's who came with the donor program worked until they almost couldn't stand up anymore to save the life of a total stranger they would never meet or see.

After nursing school I worked for one year as an RN in one of the toughest inner-city psychiatric Emergency Rooms (ER's) on the eastern side of the U.S.. Truly an unbelievable experience but just too dangerous. After seeing an advertisement for a TC position in a nursing magazine, I decided to apply and at the last minute I attached my essay along with my résumé and was interviewed and hired within a few days. I told my boss at least five times in the interview that I had no previous experience in the Intensive Care Unit (ICU) as an RN and that the majority of my past work was in the OR. It took months of training before I stopped saying that, even when out on cases. My administrator was baffled as to how I knew so much about what they did after reading the essay. I explained I had been called in as OR "on call" staff at night to do organ harvestings with their organization. We don't refer to the procedure as harvesting anymore, we call it "organ recovery." The really strange thing for me is that after doing that job for two and a half years I wouldn't change a word of that essay. It summarized perfectly the vital role that TC's silently play in having someone transplanted.

After intense training for about 12 weeks we were officially qualified to act as TC's. We had classes on donor management, brain death, legal issues facing us in transplant, hematological blood testing, organ allocation, operating room donor management, dealing with the medical examiner and, perhaps most important of all, family communication and consent. One of my coworkers said that at this stage you knew just enough to be dangerous.

We were constantly told that although doctors might be the experts on how to save people, we were the end-of-life specialists who would, as they liked to call it, "drive the bus" and ensure that the tragedy of one death would at least be mitigated somewhat through an organ transplant that allowed someone else to live. Expected to take on a leadership role in each situation, we were required to wear business professional attire while on the nursing stations and only change into scrubs when we headed into the operating room. Almost all OPO's portray the donor and the donor's family as heroes who gave graciously during the worst moment of their lives and this picture is true. But it is also important to recognize the work and dedication of the individuals who choose to work in this profession because without them, there would be no transplants.

Each OPO has hospital liaison staff who educate the medical and administrative personnel about donation. They do monthly inspections of the records of all deaths in their assigned hospitals. If they find too many "missed opportunities" — situations where the OPO was not notified of impending death — the hospital could face penalties from Medicare/ Medicaid or the Centers for Medicare & Medicaid Services (CMS), which control all Medicare and Medicaid funding in the U.S.

Most people are unaware of organ donation laws, which vary from state to state. For instance, in New Jersey if you are declared brain dead and have no family, the hospital administration has agreed that in every case the patient is classified as a potential donor and the organ donation process can move forward. In many states there is an organ donor designation on your driver's license that gives the OPO permission to move forward with or without your family's consent. We used different forms for patients with donor designation on their license. We asked the families of these donors to sign a disclosure form stating that they were aware of the wishes of the patient to donate their organs. Non-donor designated patient's families were asked to sign an actual consent form that asked for permission to transplant organs. They had to answer yes or no to the use of each organ individually.

The donor designation on a license also gives the OPO permission to send off blood tests without the family knowing the TC is even onsite. In the rare instance a patient tests positive for Hepatitis B, C or HIV the TC's are required to inform the attending physician who must then tell the family.

The TC's message was consistent: call us with all irreversible neurological injury or impending death and we will be there to assess the patient's suitability for organ donation. The only direct exceptions to this were patients with HIV and active cancer. Even Hepatitis B and C positive donor organs were used, sometimes with patients who did not already have those diseases but who could not wait any longer for a transplant or they would die. The infected organ is transplanted into the recipient and blood tests called viral loads are run to see how much of the active virus the donor had. The recipient is then treated with the appropriate antiviral medications. We evaluated a large number of elderly donors daily as well as young ones, usually those who had had hemorrhagic strokes or suffered from hypoxia, a lack of oxygen or trauma. Many patients were Coumadin users (a commonly prescribed blood thinner) who hit their heads or fell, resulting in loss of blood inside the skull.

When we started, we were each given a huge duffel bag on wheels with multiple compartments packed with all the supplies needed for at least one full case from referral to the operating room. We soon learned what to keep extra of, and how to lighten the load depending on where the case was in the process. We could always spot new TC's because they carried everything with them, every time. Eventually you became more comfortable at predicting what could happen, or at least what you thought could happen, when going onsite for a case.

We were on call 48 hours at a time; if we were out on a case more than 24 hours we got a "down" day to recover. It was normal to be called out for part of the first day and then again at 6 a.m. the second day, often with no relief until around 8 a.m. the next morning unless you had a morning operating room time. Then you stayed until everything was done. My longest case lasted from when I left home on a Friday at 6 a.m. and finished my OR liver/ kidneys recovery at 2 p.m. on Saturday. When a case is moving forward there is no time for messing around, the work is constant, labs have to be drawn, lines have to be inserted, there are tests to arrange and, of course, there is the family to deal with. There is just too much at stake to change hands every 12 hours.

We were instructed to always have a change of clothes, snacks, water and spare change because sometimes all you could eat late at night came from vending machines. Many times you would find yourself starving at about 1 a.m., having barely eaten or drank all day. The schedule appeared, at first, to give us a lot of time off, but once you start you realize this is not just a job; it's a lifestyle that affects everyone around you. As well as being on call, we also had weekly meetings where cases were discussed openly among the TC's — what you did right, what you did wrong, what you will do differently next time — they called it "quarterback."

I started out as a TC thinking that donor management would be my biggest challenge since I had had no prior experience in the ICU as a RN and that family communication would come easily as I have always been able to discuss difficult topics with people. I was so wrong! After my first year on the job, I decided I would prefer even a crashing donor to any family consent conversation. To this day, I have never done anything as hard as ask someone to donate their husband's, wife's, children's or parent's organs.

This book is a compilation of my experiences during my two and a half years as a TC. It is meant to honor those incredible individuals who choose to dedicate their lives to the cause every day and do the job as professionals, with compassion and empathy. I will always consider it an honor to have worked as one of them. Hopefully this book will also raise awareness of the need for organ donation. Squelch that urban myth everywhere that the trauma team won't work as hard to save you if you have donor designation on your license. That never happens, trauma teams don't care what brought you through their doors, they try their hardest to save your life and worry about who you are later. It's what they are trained to do. We as TC's took it personally if we heard of a recipient dying before they received an organ. On average 18 people a day die waiting. I think if I was a waiting recipient I would want to know that someone was working very hard to do two things: enable the surgeon to save a life and allow a grief-stricken family to have their loved one live on in another human being. To give life, just as another has come to an end.

■

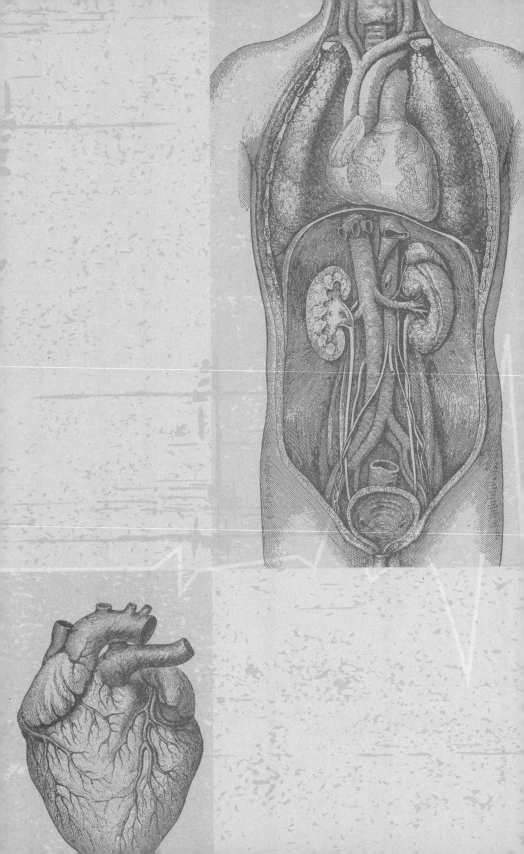

1

Brain Death

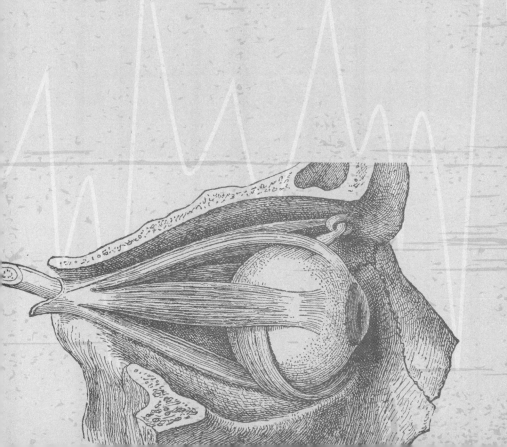

I<small>T'S IMPORTANT TO UNDERSTAND THE BRAIN DEATH PROCESS IN ORDER TO</small> completely understand the miracle of organ donation. Brain death is like being pregnant, you either are or you aren't, there is nothing in between. We know that certain injuries are more likely to lead to brain death than others. The brain is soft and easily pushed aside by blood or fluid in the skull. The patient could have a spontaneous bleed, a hemorrhagic stroke, a collection of fluid from an area deprived of oxygen or, of course, trauma. The skull is an enclosed space and the brain, fluid and spaces need to be in perfect balance for us to function, even a small collection of fluid or hydrocephalus can cause obvious, sometimes frightening, symptoms. We were trained to know how brain death happens so we knew how to explain it when we talked to the family. The moment when a patient actually becomes brain dead is when the brain is pushed so far down into the skull it literally slides through the foramen magnum, which is the hole in the bottom of our skulls where the brain and brain stem connect. This is called herniation and it is the most common time for a patient to become unstable; realize though we are talking about a transition to brain death, not saving the patient's life.

I was on a case far away from home and far away from any other Transplant Coordinators coming to my rescue. The donor's daughter had waited almost three days for her mother to progress to brain death when I was paged due to the patient's blood pressure dropping, the first sign the patient may be herniated. I rushed back into the room and found the daughter literally praying that a merciful, non-prolonged end would come for her mother. Her blood pressure was starting to dip dangerously low — 100/60 to 90/50 — so I asked the Intensive Care Unit (ICU) nurse to please hang the medication that would support the blood pressure next to the bed. She kept saying, "it's right in the Pyxis," which is the computerized pharmacy system many hospitals have, but I kept insisting she hang it on the pole next to the bed. She finally agreed and it wasn't a minute later that the mother's blood pressure totally dropped. The last thing you want to happen is have the patient code or go into cardiac arrest and, if it was going to happen, it would be at this point. What we call a code in the medical field can be loss of a heartbeat, a loss of heart rhythm or loss of blood pressure. It is extremely important that an organ donor's organs receive all the blood and oxygen they can while in a dying body. Given this, when you know a patient is irreversibly brain injured and they are progressing to brain death, you do not want them to have a cardiac arrest. Thankfully the nurse had finally listened to me just before it happened so we were able to get the mother through it and she lost all reflexes, resulting in brain death. The pressure of having a family who wants this to happen and is actually in the room as you give directions on how much and what drugs to give is unbelievable.

People have a misconception that brain death is like being in a coma. It is not at all like a coma — unless you have been given a paralytic agent, anyone, even in a coma, will still have their protective reflexes. These are the last reflexes that remain functioning and the reflexes that are individually tested before brain death is pronounced. If someone pokes you in the eye with something you should blink, if someone puts something down your throat you should gag or cough, if they shine a light in your eyes your pupils should constrict or shrink, if they roll a pen firmly over your cuticles you should draw back your hand in response to the pain. None of these reflexes are present if someone is brain dead. Declaring someone brain dead is a very specific process that is consistent but also allows some hospitals minor differences. They can do two brain death exams and an apnea test if the donor is stable. An apnea test consists of disconnecting the ventilator at the endotracheal tube for a period of about five minutes. We say that a patient "passed" the apnea test if they did not take a breath and "failed" if they breathed. Or they can do what's called a confirmatory study, which would be a cerebral blood flow study followed by one exam and always an apnea test.

To pronounce someone brain dead requires two different physicians to certify the information is consistent. They confirm that the patient is within the normal ranges for things that could potentially mask reflexes. The patient must respond in the same way for each reflex tested when both physicians go through the exam, usually 24 hours apart. The form in almost every hospital has two columns and they must certify that the following items are stable or "within normal limits": no electrolyte imbalances can be present since elevated sodium can mask reflexes, no paralytics or sedatives can be present and if the patient was given something like phenobarb they need to draw blood to be sure it is all gone from the system. It is common for brain-injured patients to be placed in a pentobarb or phenobarb coma. Patients are frequently placed by their doctors into a drug-induced coma to rest the brain and body — it slows the inflammatory process and keeps the brain from swelling so much after an injury.

The patient's acid/base blood levels must be stable for the apnea test to be correct. There were many times that we spent hours trying to correct an arterial blood gas level to do the apnea test either by increasing sodium bicarb or adjusting the respiratory rate on the ventilator. The rate on the ventilator corresponds to the number of times the vent will breathe for you per minute. How much CO_2 the patient is blowing off or retaining can dramatically affect a blood gas level. Respiratory therapists are an integral part of this process and if they are not "on board" it can make life difficult for the TC onsite. The patient has to be "normothermic," meaning having a normal body temperature of 98.6°F, because a low body temperature can mask reflexes. Each criteria on the form has a range of normal values that the patient needs to be within to be legally brain dead and by signing it, the doctor is certifying they are within that range. Lab tests are completed to certify someone is within normal range, for example, the normal sodium level is between 135 and 145 mEq/L in our blood. The brain death exam paperwork, usually the first page of at least two, asks if the patient has electrolytes within normal limits — the main ones being sodium and potassium because they make our heart muscles contract. Once that has been established they can begin the first exam to test the reflexes mentioned earlier: cough/gag, corneal reflex, pupillary reflex, withdraw from pain and the "cold calorics," which is ice water in the ear. I once had a neurologist tell me cold calorics could "wake the dead." The doctors also check for something called "doll's eyes," and then finally the respiratory drive or effort. Doll's eyes were named after those old-fashioned baby dolls whose eyes rolled around. If a patient is brain dead the eyes will roll around when the head is moved side to side. Fewer medical students and residents today are familiar with what those dolls were like so you date yourself if you can remember them.

I did see a patient respond to the cold caloric test one time and their eyes slowly drifted toward the side where the ice water was placed. Of course, I also saw a group of residents do this test and not hold the eyelids open. I pointed out to them the patient's blood pressure was rising as soon as they squirted the water in, so the patient was clearly not dead. I also found a resident looking up brain death exams on his iPhone while he did the first round of tests — I thought at least he would get it right. It was not uncommon to give the full gamut of exams and have the patient take a breath during the apnea test. Most hospitals take the patient off the ventilator for five to 10 minutes and then draw another arterial blood gas sample to confirm the CO_2 level went as high as it should. If the level goes as high as 60 and you don't take a breath, you're dead. Some policies state the CO_2 only has to rise 20 points from the starting point, some give an actual number it must reach. If you wait six minutes and the patient takes a single breath at five and a half minutes, you have to start all over from scratch, back to first exam. If they don't use a confirmatory study, which is a nuclear medicine test that "confirms" the patient has no blood flow to the brain, exams are usually done between 12 and 24 hours apart. Some pediatric policies have as long as 48 hours between exams. If the doctors decide to do a cerebral blood flow study, which more and more doctors are choosing to do, they can do an apnea test immediately following the cerebral blood flow study and pronounce the patient brain dead.

A cerebral blood flow study is pretty straightforward. An isotope is injected into the arterial system flowing up to the brain and when you see the actual pictures on the CT scan, the head has what's called an "empty skull" — you can easily see where the face and neck have blood flow and the skull is black. We would sometimes use those pictures to help a family understand what had happened and why the person was brain dead. What we knew for sure is that no one is ready to talk about donating a loved one's organs unless they first and foremost understand the patient is dead — not sleeping, not sedated, not in a coma — dead.

Once a patient was pronounced dead and we had either donor designation or consent from the family, the TC could take over medical management of the donor and act like a physician. Brain death allows nurses to work outside the Nurse Practice Act, which varies by state and dictates that a nurse can't do anything without a doctor's orders.

Once they finish the apnea testing, the patient is given a time of death. That time is like your time of birth, it will never change, even though the patient is kept on a ventilator until cross clamp in the operating room. There isn't another time given when the heart stops or the patient stops breathing. Cross clamping is when a large vascular clamp is placed across both the aorta and vena cava in the abdominal area. The aorta is the largest artery carrying oxygenated blood to the body and the vena cava is the largest vein carrying blood back to the heart and lungs to get oxygen. The time of death is precisely when the final apnea test result comes back and the physician signs the death note in the chart and brain death paperwork. The time of death was always a crucial piece of information but many times we found out that no one actually told the family the patient was dead. Many doctors and residents wanted to be the one to ask the family to allow organ donation and to hear that "yes," but we strongly discouraged doctors from asking that as it could be perceived as a conflict of interest, especially in the inner cities where many often believe that patients are not always saved because doctors want to get their organs. We would request that doctors not use terms like "passed away," "no longer with us" and, worst of all, "expired." It's interesting how healthcare providers have no problem using the word "expired" as if people are food that went bad, but cannot use the word "dead." Don't misunderstand me, the first few times you use the word "dead" with a grieving family it barely comes out, you have to almost force it off your tongue.

Typically the TC would be involved in this entire process from start to finish. We were ultimately responsible if something wasn't documented correctly. It is a crushing feeling when you've worked more than 24 hours to get someone transplanted and it all almost crashes due to a missed check off or signature. Some of the inner-city trauma centers were so used to us being there that they would literally ask the TC how they wanted the patient pronounced. At times we would opt for two exams and give the family 24 hours to come to grips with the tragedy. Other times, if we knew a donor could not be stable for very long we would opt for the quicker route. I always felt one of the toughest and emotionally draining things to do was sit in an ICU all night in the background watching the entire family file in to say their goodbyes, or watch a spouse in a bedside vigil all the way to pronouncement.

It was always a complicated procedure with many, many opportunities for things to get screwed up. In one case I worked for 36 hours to get pronouncement. The donor was a 42-year-old female who was just crossing the street in the city when she was run down by a van. The whole case was a challenge. The estranged husband and 18-year-old daughter were devastated but willing to wait and see if she progressed to brain death. This by far is one of the hardest things we helped families through, if we could. This family really wanted something positive to come of the tragedy so they waited and she did finally progress. As I was updating all my lab reports early in the morning the pronouncing physician snuck in to sign the death note. This was a hand-written note on a blank "progress note" that specified the time and date of death. This final paperwork was filled out by the chief of neurosurgery at one of the most prestigious medical schools in the world who had written the brain death policy, yet he forgot to sign one small part, which made the whole transplant process unravel in an overwhelmingly devastating manner. I was the one blamed because after working over 36 hours, the last 25 without any sleep, I did not "hold his hand" while he signed paperwork that he had drafted. I delivered my letter of resignation after that case, knowing I was totally burned out emotionally and no longer able to be as effective as I needed to be. That was after two and a half years as a TC, that taught me more than I ever could have imagined about life, death and medicine.

■

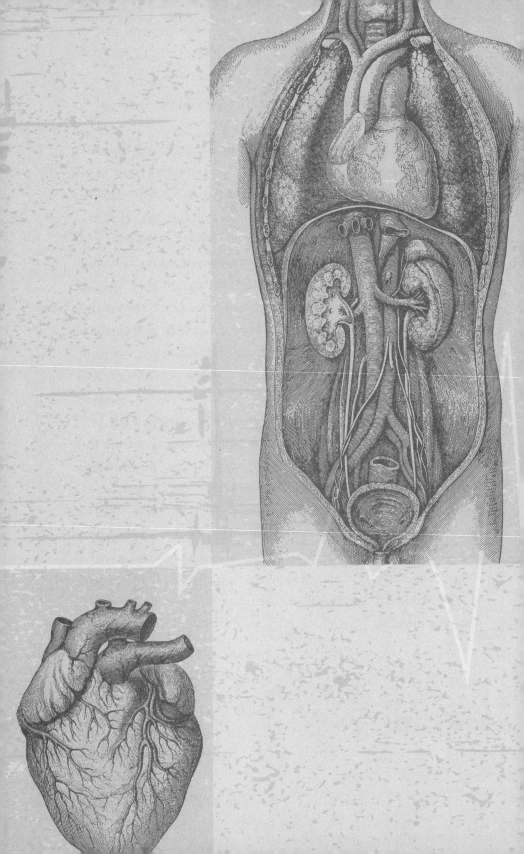

2

How to be a Transplant Coordinator

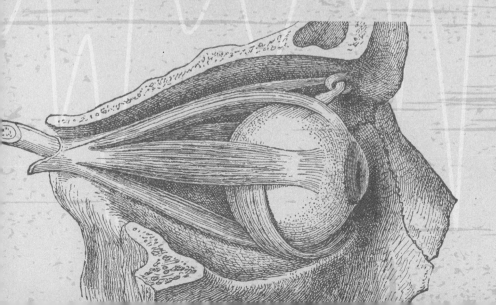

A TYPICAL DAY ON CALL STARTED AT 6 A.M. AND ENDED AT 6:00 A.M. 48 hours later. So many things can happen during those 48 hours that one of my bosses once said to me, "you're going to be in so many places today you will feel like you have multiple personalities." When you interview for a position as Transplant Coordinator they tell you at least 10 times that you should *expect* to be out on call at least 24 hours straight, with no break and no sleep. Like many people in the healthcare field I had worked some very long shifts. I spent the first 16 years of my career in the Operating Room (OR) and we frequently worked either until the surgery was done or until someone came to scrub you out, which at times could be many hours. You can't leave the OR unless someone comes to scrub you out, meaning they complete a full surgical scrub (in those days it was 10 minutes for first case of the day and three minutes in between cases), come in, gown and glove, count all sharps and sponges and then you can go. One of my favorite general surgeons used to say "you can't die from being tired," which truly did not help when you were exhausted. So I thought to myself, it can't be that bad. I completely underestimated how demanding it would be. Unless you have done it, you have no idea how bad it can really be. Working 24 hours straight makes you delirious just when you need to be at the top of your game. Many times that 24-hour shift ends with the donor in the OR, which can be the most stressful and important time and yet you are the most exhausted.

It is also very difficult to control your emotions when you are that tired so our hospital liaison staff often had to return to the unit or OR a few days later and clean up any messes the TC had created in dealing with the staff. I spent more than one and a half days on a case once where the young man's mother kept vigil at his bedside. I found myself a space at the nurse's desk at the back of the Intensive Care Unit so the mother couldn't see me — the staff had the nerve to say I was unfriendly. I have to admit though, we rarely got a talking to about such episodes, our administrators had all done this job and knew how hard it could be.

After I made it through the interview process there was a six-week training period that included two weeks of classes, followed by four brutal weeks of being on call everyday. We were sent all over the place to get as much experience with other TC's as possible. The first two weeks of training is all theory, taught by a combination of administrators and senior TC's with seven hours of classes for 10 days. Some of the subjects taught were about brain death and the legal issues facing TC's. We learned about hematology testing and how to explain the diseases they tested for, how to read the results, how to report those results to the surgeons and which results mean a donor is actively sick with something like Hepatitis B or C. The only results that immediately excluded a possible donor were HIV and current cancer, with the rare exception of a few cancerous brain tumors where we were able to confirm that the cancer had not spread anywhere else in the body. I even saw a donor test positive for syphilis (all donors are tested for this) but we gave her antibiotics and had her organs transplanted. There are certain viruses and diseases that are potentially dangerous to the recipient, like fungal infections or blood infections (septicemia). We stayed far away from those, of course, but not before a TC has spent numerous hours working like a detective and calling infectious disease transplant specialists at all hours of the day or night.

Legal issues were constantly coming up when evaluating a donor. We accessed the Department of Motor Vehicles (DMV) before going to the hospital to find out if the patient's driver's license indicated they wished to be an organ donor. Signing the form is considered "first person consent" and it holds more weight than any other person's consent because it comes directly from you. We had to know many things when faced with legal issues, especially the rights of the family, how a living will impacts the process and what to do if the donor has no next of kin. I once had to call Sing Sing prison, New York, to inquire about a homeless man without living relatives who had spent 20 years of his life there — his liver was successfully transplanted.

Living wills meant that we were frequently faced with the following scenario: the patient is severely brain injured and has signed the donor designation on his or her license but also has a living will that the family wants to honor. The problem is that many times, in order to let a patient progress to brain death, the patient needs to be given oxygen with a ventilator and have their blood pressure supported with medications and fluids for up to 72 hours. This is necessary to prevent the heart from stopping. I know this is hard to understand, but basically you can progress to brain death, given the right circumstances, without your heart ever stopping and that was exactly what we were trying to accomplish. As long as a patient is given oxygen their heart will usually continue to beat, assuming there are no other problems like electrolyte imbalances or severe blood loss. We had extensive training in what common problems we would have with brain-injured patients, like gunshot wounds to the head almost always causing problems with blood clotting. So going into a case with a gunshot wound you knew a few things before you even got there, such as that the patient will have lost and been given a very large amount of blood, crossmatched and uncrossmatched. These patients were usually too unstable to get through the brain death exams so many times we would only get liver and kidneys, and things would move very quickly. On the opposite end we had many stroke patients, hemorrhagic strokes or "bleeds" that progressed quicker to brain death than embolic strokes or "blockages." If the brain is bleeding there is nowhere for the blood to go because of the skull. So in that limited space, if the pressure created inside the skull but above the brain is not relieved surgically by either drilling a hole into the skull or taking out a flap of the skull temporarily, the brain will be pushed down to the base of the skull and eventually out through the opening that leads to the spinal cord. Once that happens no intervention will reverse the damage.

Instead of honoring the patient's wish to be an organ donor, families choose to honor the clause in the living will that says the patient is not to be put on life support. Depending on the severity of the brain injury, brain death could occur immediately or at any time within the 72-hour range. We learned that if they did not progress to brain death in that time, they usually would not and sometimes the patient would remain in a vegetative state with no meaningful recovery unless the family chose to take them off life support. I had the very rare opportunity one day to actually speak to a patient inquiring about this subject. I was at the office fixing some charts and restocking my bag when I was asked to speak to someone who had called our 1-800 number with questions. I picked up the line and introduced myself, the caller told me she was a Registered Nurse, in her mid 50's, just had a recent heart attack, her third one in two years. She was in the process of making her living will and asked specifically how it would impact her wish to be a donor. After some discussion we both agreed that the problem could be avoided by adding a simple statement like, "I do not want to be artificially resuscitated or given life-sustaining medications; the only exception is to preserve the opportunity for organ donation."

It is a very rare opportunity to be a donor. Only 1% to 2% of all people who die can be a donor and when you remove all the people who will not give their consent, the number of possible donors is even less. We are often asked whether the Organ Procurement Organization (OPO) can move forward even if the family does not wish to honor the patient's decision to be a donor. In other words, if the patient says "yes" on the license and the family says "no." I always say there are two answers to that question: what we are legally allowed to do and what we actually did. We are absolutely legally allowed to move forward with or without family approval but most OPO's, including the one I worked for, will not go against the family's wishes, it's not worth the negative publicity. That usually means a TC will have a long discussion with the family to find out why the family was refusing to honor the patient's wishes. Many times the refusal was based on either a lack of understanding of brain death or some myth the family believed, that we are like body snatchers. Once we figured out what the obstacle was we could deal with it — sometimes we got them to change their minds, sometimes we didn't.

The brain death class was an entire day that included other subjects about the clinical testing and legal implications. In the U.S. there is the Nurse Practice Act, which says a nurse can't initiate treatment without orders from a physician. Brain death allowed us to operate outside that restriction so we were able to function more like critical care physicians than nurses. We had an entire class on dealing with medical examiners because we had to get clearance from them for every donor. We needed to know about different jurisdictions, for example, if an accident occurs in one county but the patient dies in a hospital in a different county, which medical examiner do we call? We had a class on Human Leukocytic Antigen (HLA) typing (how to match hearts and kidneys) and how the recipient "list" operates, a class on tissue donation, donor assessments and dealings with hospital pathologists for biopsies. Of course there was "Consent I, II and III" and then two days of donor management. This stuff was way harder than anything we took in nursing school.

After two weeks of training we were given an on-call bag and shown how to pack it with everything we would need for a case. The bag had everything from extra charts, blood tubes, tissue packs for matching or "typing" kidneys and hearts, to handmade memory boxes for donor families and little envelopes that had printed "a wisp of hair" on the front for when a family member wanted a lock of hair as a keepsake. Each memory box was decorated with pressed flowers on the outside and contained a framed area for a picture and a smaller box to hold jewelry or keepsakes from their loved one. Once a donor was consented we would give the box to the family and explain what it was. We were taught how to read the call schedule (this almost needed its own class), assigned pagers, cell phones, laptops, corporate Visa cards and cars with Donate Life plates.

At first, we were sent out with an experienced TC. If there's a donor heading to the OR you will be going too; if there is a TC out all night moving things forward you will be planted right next to them. I remember a funny experience during training with one of my very favorite TC's. Sometime around 4 a.m. we were both so delirious that she fell asleep right at the nurse's station desk and started talking out loud about purple bubbles. I was so tired it didn't even register that she wasn't making sense. During this training time you are exposed to all different parts of the process, so you may start out in the city sitting in on a consent conversation, then go to another place to do allocation of the organs to be transplanted, then to yet another to get into the OR for an organ recovery.

There was a rural hospital that had a reputation for being very difficult with us, making the TC's sit in the conference room and never allowing them on the unit even after they had consent from a patient for a transplant. On my very last day of the grueling four weeks of on-call training I was sent to this hospital. It's over a four-hour drive and when I arrived I found the TC sitting in the conference room as expected. We began evaluating a male in his 40s who had suffered a spontaneous intracranial bleed. There's some wild story about the patient's brother who was there earlier in the day claiming to be a shaman. He said he was able to transport himself through time and may make an appearance as an apparition to check on his brother. Whoa.

We were responsible to get the patient pronounced brain dead, allocate his organs to recipients and set up the operating room. The process was going along fine, pronouncement was easy and we were quietly allocating on our laptops when the door burst open and a nurse and a resident who were very upset exclaimed, "your patient just kicked his right leg, he's not dead!" When we got to the patient's room there were more staff members watching and, sure enough, the patient kicked his right leg up about 12 inches off the bed and then immediately lifted his right arm. The neuro resident was very upset. The TC started explaining that it's a spinal reflex, not purposeful movement, and that the two are like night and day. It was obvious that we had a problem only the attending physician could fix when she would arrive in the morning. The pronouncing physician, a female neurologist in her early 60s, came to find us when her residents filled her in on the overnight drama. The TC was in a delirious ramble trying to explain everything from the shaman who could supposedly transport himself to the kicking leg. Every few sentences the doctor said "uh huh" until she suddenly asked, "I only want to know one thing, why aren't you in the OR yet?" As we left we overheard the doctor refreshing her staff on spinal reflexes.

This is a good time I think to explain how the organ transplant process works. The hospital calls the office with a "referral," a patient who has been admitted with some kind of irreversible brain injury. The injury could be caused by a gunshot, a bleed in the brain or hypoxia if they went too long without oxygen. The office takes basic demographic information and pages the Clinical Phone Coordinator on call (we all did this job on a regular basis — 24 excruciating hours) who must return the call to the hospital in five minutes. She calls the hospital to speak to either the patient's nurse, the resident or the attending physician and finds out the following things: the patient's date of birth, age, sex, history of present illness or what brought them into the hospital, any significant past medical history, the current neurological status, what reflexes are present, current vital signs, any IV medications being given to support the blood pressure, what is the family situation and who is making decisions and, finally, what is the hospital's plan or course of action at the present time.

Once the Clinical Phone Coordinator has all this information, she calls the office and has them check with the DMV to see if the patient has requested that his organs be donated on the driver's license. Once that information is gathered she calls the Administrator on Call, who decides which TC is going to be assigned to the case. The Clinical Phone Coordinator then pages the TC, who has a maximum of 30 minutes to get on the road. Once in the car you call the Administrator on Call to let them know you're on the way, then you call the hospital unit and give them an estimated time of your arrival and instructions to call if there are any changes in the patient's condition before you arrive.

We also had a class on the OR experience. Our building had two complete operating suites capable of doing a multi-organ recovery if a donor was stable enough to be moved (which most are not). This class was taught by three TC's who were former paramedics. I felt the whole thing was silly. They spent more time grandstanding and pretending to be rogue surgeons than they did actually teaching. I spent 16 years in the OR handing instruments to surgeons and this display was embarrassingly inaccurate. What I did realize was that you could work in many different areas of medicine but your equipment and supplies are pretty much the same everywhere. The OR staff were notoriously unforgiving to people who didn't know what they were doing. We used to say surgeons could smell fear and OR nurses ate their young (I say that with love former OR coworkers. I was right there along with you.). It could feel like a three-ring circus when you had multiple teams coming for multiple organs, each team having at least a couple of surgeons who were trained in transplant and each one coming by different modes of transportation. My first organ recovery as a TC was in a small rural hospital. All the staff wanted to watch so they lined up along the back wall of the room. That case had its challenges, as they all do; the problem tonight was that the lung surgeon coming via helicopter was delivered to me in a wheelchair by the air ambulance pilots, airsick from turbulence. She was a small feisty female in her 50s, known for being tough but she didn't have much to say this time. When the recipient team called with timing questions and I told them she was airsick, she freaked yelling, "Don't tell them that!" She was fine after I gave her some crackers and a cold soda, although neither improved her attitude.

The real schedule was a combination of on-call, attending meetings and educational conferences, sometimes we listened and sometimes we had to speak at area hospitals. There were four seminars a year called Donation Champion Meetings that were offered to the hospital staff involved in the organ recovery process, mostly RN's and Respiratory Therapists. They were always very popular and packed to capacity with waiting lists for cancellations. It was a day full of interesting speakers including a donor family, a couple of recipients and at least one transplant surgeon.

Once you made it through the orientation training you were presented with a certificate that certified you as a Transplant Coordinator and had your picture taken wearing a "training-graduation cap." Now you were qualified to go out on your own. The training was rough but nothing compared to being out on your own with a massive amount of responsibility on your shoulders. When all the training is complete and you have proven yourself to be relatively independent you are presented with a certificate that says you have done the following:

- Demonstrated the stamina to be awake and alert for an incredible period of time.
- Demonstrated the ability to have multiple phone conversations while simultaneously providing reasonable donor management advice.
- Demonstrated the ability to accurately complete seemingly endless

pages of donor charting, make copies and send faxes while fighting true exhaustion.

- Demonstrated the ability to subsist on only junk food, more of which you ever thought possible.
- Demonstrated the ability to drive many miles, to faraway places, despite getting lost, to facilitate life-saving organ transplants for our recipients.

When you can do this, you are officially declared a Transplant Coordinator.

■

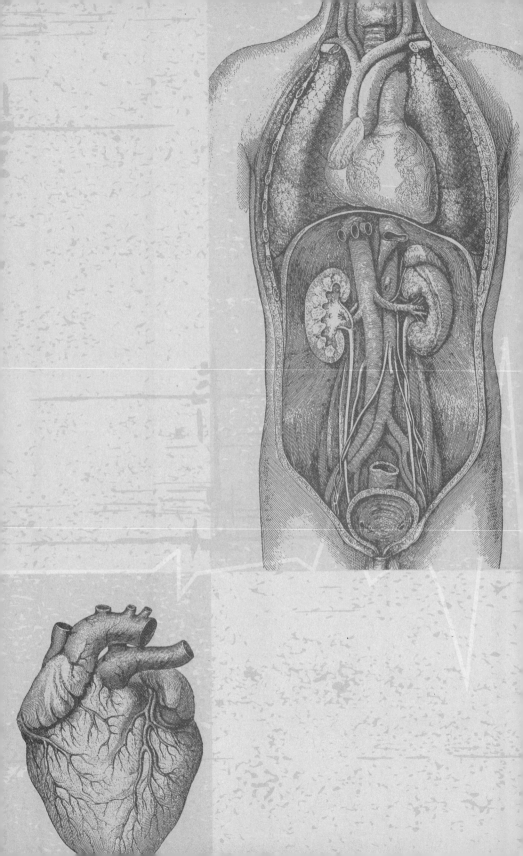

3

A Bad
Decision

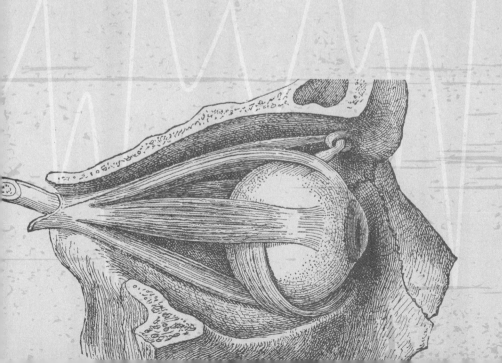

D URING ONE OF MY FIRST DAYS ON CALL I BEGAN TO REALIZE THAT THIS was the most physically, emotionally and psychologically exhausting thing I'd ever done. Whenever I felt that way I reminded myself that I was still better off than whomever I was being sent out to evaluate. That morning I was headed into the city again to evaluate a young female donor. There weren't many notes on her in our computer system and that usually means the Transplant Coordinator onsite had been very busy. That TC was called out late in the night to start the evaluation. It was his second day of call on his rotation, so instead of having to stay for more than 24 hours, I was sent to relieve him. It was a beautiful day, cold but sunny. After about an hour on the road, most of it in traffic, I arrived at the hospital and walked onto the medical Intensive Care Unit (ICU). Today, hospitals don't have only one ICU, the big ones have several and we frequented them all. I looked all over for my coworker. I knew he'd be there somewhere; we would often park ourselves in some back corner or room in the unit. We still needed to be able to see the monitors or be close by at the very least. Once the donor was pronounced or consented we would move out to the front of the room.

I found him in the lounge talking to a resident. He introduced me to the senior resident who was about to tell the family of this young girl that she has been pronounced brain dead. "Then they will be ready to talk to you," she said and walked away. My coworker ran through the important parts that I needed to know. I could read the rest in the chart later. This beautiful

26-year-old female had hung herself in her home. He didn't know a lot of details because he had not yet spoken with the family and, as usual, he had been busy all night in the background getting things ready to move forward. She was young and she was donor designated. Believe it or not, I am actually more comfortable in a situation where I come in and have to talk to the family right away instead of sitting around for hours and hours thinking about it. The resident came out, said they were ready for me and said she thinks they may know why I'm there. We had extensive training for this conversation and the Organ Procurement Organization (OPO) preferred us to stick to what we had been taught because it worked. We all spent hours in a consent workshop role-playing hundreds of possible family scenarios. I hated the role-playing. The instructors claimed that if you said something stupid in role-play there was a very high probability you would say something as stupid in front of the family. We were trained to initially be very vague about who we were and why we were there. We didn't have scrubs on and we didn't have a name badge. We were introduced as many different things like an "end of life specialist," or, "someone the healthcare team partners with in situations like these." We were taught to say we were part of the healthcare team, but I made the mistake of saying it in front a neurosurgeon once and he said in no uncertain terms that we are NOT members of the healthcare team and then told me not to use that introduction. I wasn't upset or offended, in fact my reply to him was, "You're right, I'm not a member of the healthcare team, how do you suggest I introduce myself?" I used his suggestion, "someone the healthcare team partners with in situations like these" for the rest of my time in that career, it was perfect. Neurosurgeons were one of our biggest challenges in the process mainly because most of our donors were the result of their failures. Many times the neurosurgeon is the physician who does one of the brain death exams, so you hoped any interaction with them would go well. This time I didn't have to set anything up, they were waiting for me.

Together with the bedside nurse who was quite emotional, I went into a darkened corner in the depths of the ICU. The nurse introduced me and I sat across from the young girl's mother and between her husband and father. Her young husband had his head in his hands on the table, her father was looking off in the distance somewhere, her mother, however, was looking right at me. I started out the way I was taught, asking them what they knew about what had happened. That gave me time to collect my thoughts and let me know how much of what was going on they understood. We knew that if the family didn't completely understand their loved one was dead there could be no talk of organ donation. This family knew what was going on though; they had been well informed and involved during the night as she made a turn for the worse. They told me what had transpired to get her here; she had been a vibrant, very active, young wife and mother of two daughters, two nights ago she had a fight with her husband. She was known to sometimes be a little overly dramatic and had recently started taking an antidepressant prescribed by her family doctor. They said she had threatened in the past to kill herself during emotional upheavals but it seemed to be more attention-seeking behavior than real intention.

I think it is irresponsible when a family doctor prescribes psych meds and doesn't send the person to a psychologist or counselor. Many family doctors don't understand the way psych meds work and have no idea that the risk of suicide actually increases in some people in the first few weeks of antidepressant use. Patients started on these meds should be watched closely. When a person is seriously depressed they usually lack the ability to formulate and carry through with a suicide plan. They may threaten suicide but almost never follow through with it, which only makes matters worse because then the family starts thinking their depression is all about getting attention. When I worked as a Registered Nurse in a very busy Crisis Response Unit in the inner city, which is like a psychiatric emergency room, I saw many suicide attempts that were really just to prove to the family that the person was serious about needing help. As the antidepressant kicks in during the first few weeks they have more energy and are able to focus their thoughts better, which often leads to suicide or at least an attempt.

This girl, however, made a bad decision after an argument that took her life. She had taken some prescription painkillers from a minor surgical procedure; she had a fight with her husband and said she was going upstairs to hang herself. She went into a closet and tied a belt from a robe around her neck and tied the other end around the clothes rod. Then she fell into a deep sleep from the painkillers she had taken — although this may seem hard to believe. She did not overdose herself. Her husband did not check on her, he fell asleep watching television downstairs and found her later that night when he finally went to bed. She had just enough oxygen in her system to keep her heart beating but not enough to keep her brain alive.

It was at this point that her mother looked at me and said with a straight face, "You're here to talk to us about donating her organs, aren't you?" Once the subject is out on the table it makes things a little easier, so I went right into discussing how she had indicated her wish to be a donor on her driver's license. Unfortunately, the time had come to honor her wish and give her the ability to live on in another person. They all knew she had signed the donor form on her license and accepted the opportunity to donate her organs. We went through our disclosure form and her husband, being her legal next of kin, signed all necessary paperwork to move forward. Her mother started asking me very specific questions about incisions and where they would be, she said she already knew what they would bury her in and wanted to make sure any incisions wouldn't be visible. I explained to her that if the top of her outfit was low cut the chest incision would most likely be seen, but after talking with her, she decided it was not worth limiting her daughter's gift. Her father couldn't stand it any longer and politely got up and excused himself to go sit with her, her husband followed him. I really did not know what to say to this beautiful but grieving mother. She had already allowed her son-in-law and granddaughters to move into her home because the thought of going back to the place where her daughter had died would be too much for them. She talked about what kind of person her daughter was, how she was kind and vivacious, a loving and dedicated mother to her two girls who adored her. She pulled a picture out of her purse and handed it to me across the table. It was a picture of her daughter, kneeling next to her kitchen table with a little tiara on her head and a handmade sign behind her on the table saying, "Happy Birthday Mom." I was almost overcome with the thought of not seeing my own daughters again, not feeling their hair, touching their hand or hearing them laugh. I just don't know how people find the strength to go on, especially with the loss of a child, even an adult one. No parent should have to bury their child. Her mother looked at me and asked, "Will I ever be happy again? Will I ever feel joy or peace?" I could have given her the typical answer, "oh yes, you will get past this," but that would have been a lie. Sometimes you need to talk about the tough subjects with these families because no one else will. I told her she might find happiness again someday and I was sure she would find joy in watching her granddaughters grow up, but her life would never be the same again. She appreciated my honesty and wanted me to put her daughter's picture with her chart. I promised her that everyone who came for the organ recovery would see it. We walked out to her room together.

The family asked how long they could stay and I told them they could stay with her right up until we went to the operating room if they wanted, but it was also fine to go home now. We found that many families at this point did not know what to do next and it was helpful to suggest that many families say their last goodbyes now and go home — it was almost like they could not go home until they found out that's what other families did. I still had hours and hours of work to do though. We needed to turn her kidneys back around to a normal function as soon as possible, this was done by giving drugs and IV fluids to flush the kidneys. Sometimes when a person has been "down," meaning they have been unconscious or unresponsive for an extended period of time, they go into acute renal failure. Other problems start to occur when the kidneys fail—the body starts to have electrolyte imbalances with sodium and potassium, both of which need to be within normal limits for brain death testing but frequently are out of balance due to the decrease in kidney function. Her potassium was already getting higher and so was her sodium, she was starting to retain water and swell. This condition is called "third spacing" and means that the body will hold fluids outside of the vascular system. Since the body can't get rid of the excess fluid we would give albumin to pull the fluid out of the tissues and then Lasix, which is a drug that gets rid of extra fluid. Of course, along with all that fluid goes her electrolytes.

One of the very first things we initiated with any pronounced donor was what we called T4. When the brain dies the body can no longer put out certain hormones, most importantly T3 from the pituitary gland. It's an important hormone for what is called homeostasis, which controls the overall balance of things. We gave every brain-dead donor T4 or Levothyroxine through an IV drip, the goal is to enhance the hemodynamic and metabolic stability of the donor. Thyroid hormones, T3 and T4, regulate the rate and efficiency of energy being used within the cells. Research indicates that serum thyroid hormone levels drop quickly during brain herniation and are undetectable by blood test within hours of brain death. The destruction of the hypothalamus and pituitary glands (within the brain) during herniation prevents the body from getting those hormones through the normal path. The absence of normal thyroid hormone results in diffuse metabolic injury at the cellular level, which becomes apparent in a multitude of problems and can ultimately lead to instability and organ deterioration. T4, converted to T3 by our bodies, is the preferred hormone in adults because it is inexpensive and available through most hospital pharmacies. We started the procedure out with the following cocktail of

IV boluses (a bolus is when you push a drug into the vascular system all at one time as opposed to a drip which gives a set amount of fluid or drug per minute or per hour): Levothyroxine 20 mcg, Solumedrol (a steroid) 2 g, Dextrose (sugar) 50% 50 ml, regular insulin 20 units and Vasopressin (a blood pressure supporting medication) 1 unit. They were given in rapid succession through the central IV line then followed by a drip of T4.

We had an entire page of orders we implemented as soon as we took over. For a full donor, where as many organs as possible would be salvaged, we would send the labs material to test to monitor kidney function, liver and pancreas function and lung function every four hours. We had labs we used that were outside of the hospital too. Usually there were about eight boxes with five tubes in each box; that's 40 tubes of blood. Each one had to be labeled, packed and couriered to the various transplant centers for matching. All heart donors needed an echocardiogram, which is an ultrasound of the heart, and an electrocardiogram (EKG). One of the problems was in order to evaluate the heart function you needed to get the donor off some of the blood pressure supporting medications. That process could sometimes take hours of running T4, fluids and sometimes giving blood products as well. All brain-dead donors had difficulty supporting their own blood pressure and they had a complete loss of their vasomuscular tone, affecting the heart and blood vessels. Every donor needed a urinalysis to ensure there was no active kidney or bladder infections. All females, regardless of age, needed a *Human Chorionic Gonadotropin* (HCG) pregnancy test, an increased level of HCG should only be present when you are pregnant so in postmenopausal women it can indicate a cancer. Every lung donor needed a chest X-ray and a bronchoscopy to look inside the lungs.

All that may sound simple enough, but let me give you a few common roadblocks: it's the middle of the night and you need to call in a pulmonary doctor to do the bronchoscopy, you need to call in the echo team and cardiologist to get the echo and you need to call in the cardiac catheterization team if needed. Trying to get all these people to cooperate never went smoothly. People protested because it was a donor rather than a living patient or they couldn't find the equipment they needed because it was late at night. We did exercises on the lungs to see how much we could improve them, respiratory therapy helped with this. First we had to draw an arterial blood gas, and then they change the ventilator settings for about 20 minutes and then redraw another blood gas to see what effect it had on the lungs. The respiratory therapists could change the settings to either make the patient breathe out more CO_2 or breathe in more oxygen, which directly affects the amount of acid or base in our blood. Blood gases could be very complicated and we had to know how to correct them because it was an integral part of the brain death testing.

As I was getting ready to start allocating her organs to recipients her parents decided to leave. In front of the ICU staff her father walked over to me, put his hands on my shoulders, looked me in the eyes and said, "Please ... take care of my daughter and make something good come of this." I hugged them both, assured them all I would work my hardest to give them something to hold on to, got everyone's cell phone number and promised to call her father after the organ recovery procedure in the operating room. I told them I anticipated being in the operating room by early morning and they could call me at any time.

The heart is removed first and the rest of the organs are removed in this order: lungs, liver, pancreas and kidneys. The organs have to go in this order because of timing with the recipients. Hearts and lungs can only be outside of the body for four hours maximum including travel time. The liver and pancreas can be out for about eight hours and kidneys can be outside of a living body for up to 48 hours. Once the organs are allocated we then backed them up with other recipients farther down the list, a practice that was done every time, in an effort to never have an organ go to waste. Anyone who knows a recipient who has waited for an organ transplant knows about the "false alarms." In many of these cases the patient is second or third in line, but when a rare opportunity arises they alert the patient and bring them into the transplant center immediately. Once the operating room time was set, I would need to arrange transportation for the surgical teams that collected the organs and brought them to the recipients. Transportation could at times be by helicopter, by ambulance, by limo, by chartered plane and sometimes our perfusionist picked them up. All depended on where the surgical recovery team was coming from and what they were coming to get. That night would be easy though, this girl's organs were healthy so most of the recipients were from local transplant programs. Organs were allocated to the closest patients first, especially with hearts and lungs, but that was because of timing. Then we would go into the regional and national lists. The surgeons who came from the north preferred to come by limo so they could sleep. If you are working in transplant on the donor side you never know when you will next have time to sleep. Having a healthy donor and a gracious family is a rare opportunity and one not to be missed because it's late at night or the weather is too stormy or windy to fly. All the surgical teams arrived within a few minutes of each other. As I reviewed the necessary paperwork with each team I made sure the girl's picture was right there for all to see. I kept my promise to her mother and made sure every single person involved in that room saw how beautiful she had been in life. The operating room circulating nurse got choked up when she placed the picture on the whiteboard attached to the wall. Everything went well and the case went smoothly. Five lives were saved that day due to the donor's selfless gift. Five people she didn't know — but each one someone's mother, sister, brother or spouse — will never forget her.

I had been there almost 24 hours. I finished up audiotaping the report with the office, called the Medical Examiner to let him know we were done and started my walk to the car. I still had to call her family but decided to wait until I was almost home to make that call. I drove most of the way in silence, almost as if I needed a break from thinking. I had my list of where her organs went next to me in the car with her father's cell phone number at the top of the page. I got off the highway, drove into a park where I could see the sunrise through the trees and called him. He answered on the second ring, said no he wasn't sleeping when I asked if I had woken him. He had been waiting for my call. I told him everything went great. Her right kidney and pancreas went to a 52-year-old male. Her left kidney was a perfect match for a 19-year-old female. A 32-year-old female received her liver. Both lungs went to a 51-year-old male and last but not least her precious heart went to a very sick 45-year-old male. I could hear him quietly weeping on the other end of the phone. I promised to send him a follow-up letter in a few weeks with more information about the recipients. He thanked me and said they were going to proudly display this information at her funeral. Many of us place those little organ donor words on our driver's license. None of us ever think it will be used. I felt honored to be able to fulfill her last wish.

■

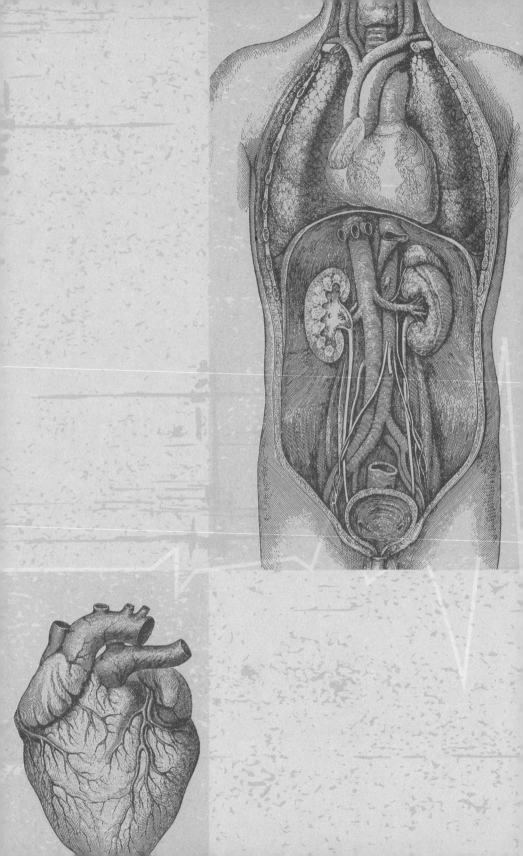

4

Donation after Cardiac Death

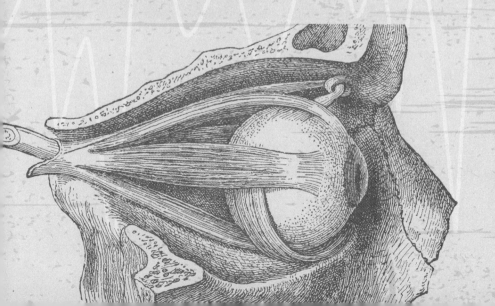

THERE ARE RARE INSTANCES WHEN THE SITUATION FORCES THE TRANS-plant Coordinator to arrange for the presence of family members in the operating room. There are two reasons to be pronounced clinically dead in the U.S.: brain death or cardiac death. The process called "Donation after Cardiac Death" (DCD) presents a very small window of opportunity for donation and the organs that can be donated are limited to just the liver and kidneys. It only happens when the donor is not brain dead but severely brain injured with no hope of meaningful recovery. Families who have a loved one in this situation are usually given two options, the first one being a tracheostomy for long-term ventilator support and a feeding tube for long-term feeding. Many families choose to do these procedures and the patient is eventually moved to a long-term care facility. We did not speak to the families of patients who made that decision, it was a one-way move off our radar.

The families who opted to withdraw life support or make the patient comfortable and let them go were the families we had to talk to, before the patient was taken off the ventilator or extubated. As a Clinical Phone Coordinator, those calls to the families made up many of the referrals you got that would go nowhere because the patients were not brain dead and were either too old or not brain injured enough to be a DCD donor. These patients were sometimes ones we had been monitoring for brain death when the Clinical Phone Coordinator made her daily calls at 5 a.m., 1 p.m. and 9 p.m.

After the family had made the decision to withdraw support, we came to talk to them. Many times the nurse at the hospital would ask us what she should tell the family to buy time for us to get there. We had many answers: tell them you need to get the morphine from the pharmacy, you need to wait until the doctor signs something or you need to get out your other patient's medications first. The last thing you wanted was to have to ask the family over the phone to donate the patient's organs. We were trained to say that it's too important of a conversation to have over the phone and could they please wait until you get to the hospital and give them an estimate of when you will arrive. Some nurses insisted on telling the family that a TC was coming, which never helped the situation.

I had many families say they wished organ donation had been made an option right at the start, but usually once I explained to them that it would be considered unethical by some people because they would think we were asking them to withdraw life support so that we could take the organs, they understood.

If the family was interested in pursuing donation we could ask them to wait and see if brain death would occur. If this was going to happen it was usually within 48 to 72 hours after the injury if there had been no intervention to stop the bleeding or to relieve pressure inside the skull. The families that chose to wait for this to happen always struggled through the whole time and a TC would be present every day just to talk with the family. Some families couldn't take the emotional pain and would decide they wanted to withdraw life support.

If the final decision was to withdraw support, we changed the case to DCD. The process was explained to the family like this: the Intensive Care Unit (ICU) nurses and doctors would come to the operating room along with the patient, the same as if the withdraw was happening on their unit. We did not offer the family a chance to come into the operating room with them but many times the family asked and we had to admit that we could arrange it. The ICU team would give whatever medications they use at their facility for withdraw of care, usually morphine. The TC will have nothing to do with this process, they will sit and record the vital signs during that time and there will be a second TC who will be with the family.

The first thing that had to be done was a respiratory drive assessment, a measurable test to see how the patient would do once the ventilator was removed. We informed the attending physician and had a little meeting with the resident, nurse and respiratory therapists assigned to the patient. We wanted to mimic extubation (taking a patient off artificial respiration) as closely as we could without actually extubating or causing instability. Respiratory Therapy would need to do a test called a Negative Inspiratory Force (NIF) that measures the negative pressure that helps draw air into the lungs when we take a breath. I've been told this is uncomfortable for the patient, making them feel like they are breathing through a straw. I even had one patient, who was not as severely brain damaged as we thought, who cried every time they did a NIF. Our "respiratory drive" is the combined effort of voluntary movements we make to breathe. So once everyone was in the room, including family, sometimes we disconnected the ventilator and documented how the patient's vital signs changed. Depending on the severity of brain damage, the heart rate and oxygen saturation may change quickly or slowly. If we could be relatively sure the patient would die within 60 to 90 minutes and the family had consented, we would move forward. It takes a few hours to get the liver and kidneys allocated and the team of surgeons to the hospital and there's a ton of communication that needs to take place with the operating room staff. Liver and kidneys are the only organs that can be recovered in a cardiac death patient and there are age restrictions, no one over the age of 45-50. Talking to the Operating Room (OR) staff before and during one of these cases is really important. They are people who are not accustomed to death; OR staff and surgeons will make every effort to ensure a patient does not die in the OR and I have even seen CPR done until the patient is in the ICU. Then they stop and call time of death. Surgical staff probably have never seen the withdraw process that occurs on the units daily, anesthesia staff at almost every hospital would not even come into the room. Add to that the strong opinions and personalities of the OR staff, and the request to bring family and you have yourself a DCD.

The most important thing to make these cases successful is communication with the OR staff, the ICU staff and the family. We would do our best to prepare them for what they would see, what they could and couldn't touch and tell them that they must leave the OR no more than five minutes after death is declared. The ICU staff that worked in the OR needed to know a few things as well. They needed to make sure they had all the medications necessary because once we were in the OR the only people with access to things like morphine was anesthesia and they wanted no part in a DCD. The resident who pronounced the patient dead based on cardiac death could not leave until the process was completed, so they needed to ensure that there was another doctor to cover for them in the event of an emergency or code somewhere else in the hospital.

We also explained in detail what each of the TC's would do: one would be with the family for support and the other would be recording vital signs until death and communicating with the surgeons who would be waiting outside the room. The surgeons knew the rules, no looking through the windows or coming in until the TC came to get them five minutes after death, to ensure there is no auto-resuscitation. Everyone is given a clear and consistent message: the TC's would not get involved in the actual withdraw of life support process, which included the extubation or removal of the breathing tube and the sedation of the patient to an acceptable level of comfort.

Once everything was ready, the patient, ICU team and primary TC headed to the OR while the other TC stayed with the family. If the family would be going into the OR they got changed or covered their clothes and hair and put masks on and then waited until someone came to get them. In the OR the perfusionist would break up sterile bags of ice with a mallet; this person came for every organ recovery, sometimes they would bring a surgical team near our office with them if they came to recover an organ. They were responsible for bringing the flushing and storage solutions, boxes for transporting organs, helping the surgical teams flush the body and organs with a sugary, very cold preservation fluid and sometimes even transporting the kidneys and/or liver to their destinations. Our perfusionists were awesome, and they also did what were called "fly outs" with transplant teams in our region. That was when a local transplant team was flying somewhere to get an organ for a local recipient, they would fly with them and help pack up and transport the organ back safely. Like I've said there were procedures and regulations for everything including how an organ was packed in a bag or container, covered in ice, placed in a bag, then a box and taped closed, of course all after being labeled multiple times and verified with the TC. The OR staff were busy setting up instruments on sterile tables, and counting their instruments. I have been on that side of the table as a surgical technologist and we didn't count sharps or sponges for a donor recovery, but we did count instruments and there were hundreds for a multi-organ recovery. The surgeons got into their scrubs, came in the room, gown and glove to prep the patient and cover him with sterile drapes. The sterile drapes were then covered with an extra set of sterile and then unsterile drapes and finally a warm blanket, the patient was positioned on the OR table on their back with one arm tucked at the side and the other arm extended out on an armboard so the family could touch them or hold their hand. The OR, which is usually pretty lively and loud, was solemn and quiet out of respect for the donor's family. During the withdraw of life support the ICU nurse had the authority to give as much morphine as needed to make the patient comfortable. The breathing tube was removed and we suction out the mouth if needed. The family was then brought into the room and guided to sit next to the patient. There was always palpable tension in the room at that point.

What happened next sometimes was quick and sometimes slow, but if death did not occur within 60 to 90 minutes the patient would be moved back to a regular room where they would continue to be given comfort care until they died. The family was well prepared for this by the TC's. I have seen this unpleasant situation where the patient is moved back to a regular room to die unfold three times. One of them when I was a surgical tech in the OR and two while I was a TC. All three patients took a few days to die.

If death did occur in the OR within the 90-minute timeframe the family was escorted out and, following a strictly enforced five-minute waiting period, the surgeons came in, uncovered the patient and made an incision all the way down the abdomen. We waited the five minutes in case of something called "auto resuscitation," a rarely seen phenomenon where the heart can start beating again for a few seconds. Things moved very quickly at that point. Large bore cannulas or tubes were placed into the aorta and vena cava (the two largest blood vessels in the body) to pump cold preservation fluid into the kidneys and liver and basins of sterile ice were dumped into the abdominal cavity. The liver had to be removed as quickly as possible and the kidneys came out last. The kidneys may not even have been assigned to recipients at that point, but they would stay out of the body for up to 48 hours.

I had one very interesting DCD case at a very large hospital that was a woman from India who went into liver failure while here visiting with her two sons. She received a liver transplant and was doing well until, while in physical therapy at the Rehab, she fell and hit her head. She never regained consciousness. It was very difficult for us to even get to speak with the sons because the doctors were being protective of the situation. No one expected the sons to say yes. The staff had allowed her hemoglobin to decrease to 7.0

(a normal female should be between 9.0 and 11.0) so we would need to have given the patient a considerable amount of blood if they did say yes. I was with a senior TC and I was thankful she led the conversation with the sons that ended in them saying yes.

There was lots of conversation about their culture and the way in which they handle death. They wanted to bring a few items into the OR during the withdraw process. It started with a Buddhist chant on a CD that played over and over in the OR. They brought out a beautiful tapestry in vibrant colors and gently draped it across their mother's body and one son placed a small pile of rice in the palm of her hand. They explained to us that all these items were to help her into the afterlife, the music to show her the path, the rice in case she was hungry and the tapestry so she was dressed up for her exit from this world and entrance into the next. The OR staff respected their culture and allowed her sons to say goodbye to their mother in their own way. She was able to save three lives that day by donating her kidneys and the liver that she had received herself only a few weeks ago.

I was also involved in a case like this that didn't go so well. This time the patient was positioned the same way on the table with one arm tucked under the sheet next to the body and the other on an armboard near the family. The nurse didn't realize until the family was present that the arm with the IV was tucked in the draw sheet next to the body so she could not get to it when the patient needed more morphine. The patient struggled to breath for most of the time in the OR. Time moved much too slowly, because the family was so dedicated we waited the whole 90 minutes. The patient was moved up to another room and died a few days later.

There was a case that I was not personally involved in but it was talked about in great detail in many meetings by the TC's who were involved. A woman contacted our office asking about donating her husband's organs. He was suffering from Lou Gehrig's disease (ALS), which causes a decline in voluntary muscle movements in the patient, including breathing, until they are in what is referred to as a "locked in" state where the patient cannot move anything. They can't even blink their eyelids but it is believed they are mentally intact. Patients are hopefully encouraged by their physician to make end-of-life decisions before they get to that stage.

At one of our area hospitals there was an entire unit of these patients, some of whom were admitted literally to withdraw ventilator support and make them comfortable. The huge difference for us was that these patients made the decision to terminate life support themselves — for themselves. They would indicate very specifically when they wanted to be removed from the ventilator. Breathing is voluntary. If you have lost the ability to move your diaphragm you cannot breathe. A woman and her husband had made the decision to take him off the ventilator, he was in his mid-40s and had been a very active, dynamic, loving father of two young children. He was only able to communicate now through a computer program that turned the letter he focused on into a typed letter or word. He was still able to move his eyes and blink, but that was all and he knew his time was very limited. They requested a TC come to their home, where the patient was living, and talk about donation after cardiac death.

Two of our best TC's went out to their home to discuss the opportunity, one male and one female. This was a very unique experience, the patient himself answered the questions in the medical social questionnaire and he gave consent and allowed any preliminary bloodwork to be drawn at his home. He was admitted to the ALS unit a week later, on a day the patient had chosen, in the afternoon and the TC's met him there. They had lines to place and surgeons to talk to but they allowed the patient to set the OR time. He was choosing the time he would die. The patient also communicated that he did not want any sedation until they actually were about to extubate. He said he wanted to remember everything. The night before the withdraw his wife brought his two young children in to say goodbye. When the TC's told us about this case at our morning meeting they were crying and so was everyone else. They told us how, when the kids were there, the TC's went off by themselves and ended up outside watching the sunset, quietly supporting each other and appreciating the beauty of something so simple.

The next morning they asked the patient if he was sure this was what he wanted. He blinked once, which meant yes. The wife, the TC's, the nurses and the doctor in charge of the ALS unit started down to the OR. They positioned the patient on the OR table, draped him like we always did but left his face uncovered. One of the TC's noticed the patient continued to focus on his wife, looking at her like he didn't want to ever forget her face, and he was blinking three times in a row over and over. She was overcome with emotion when she realized the patient was telling his wife "I love you" with each set of three blinks. They played his favorite music and his wife never left his side as the doctor injected the morphine into the IV, the endotracheal tube was removed and he died. His liver and kidneys were successfully transplanted into three people. There was no hope for the patient; ALS is a terminal illness with no cure. When there was no hope, we were there. Helping the patient to leave a legacy; a part of him lived on in another person.

■

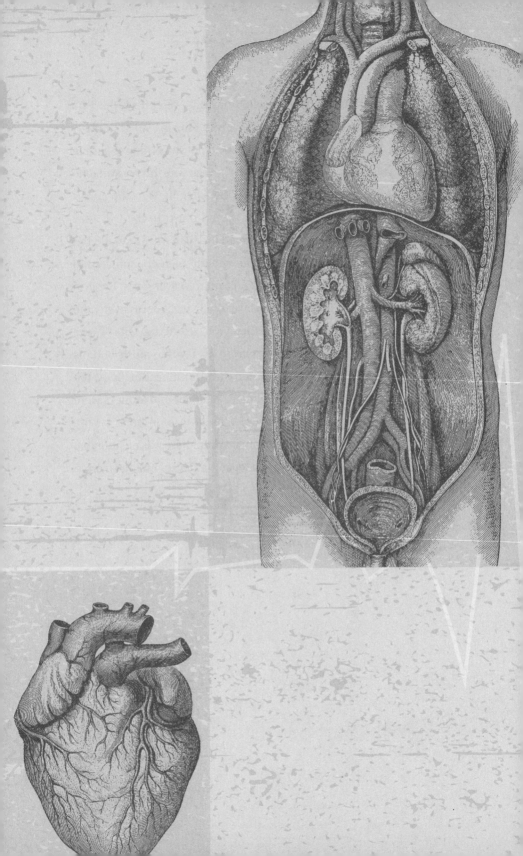

5

Pablo

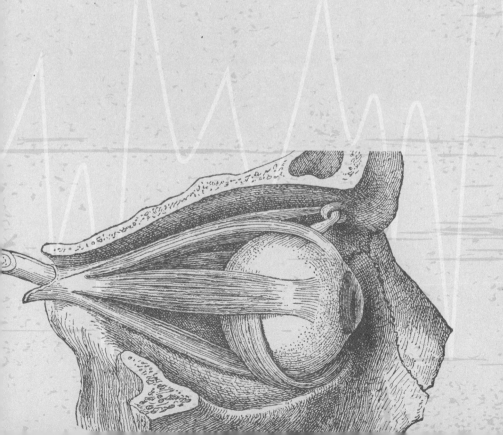

I WAS ON MY WAY TO ANOTHER CITY HOSPITAL TO SEE ANOTHER DRUG OVER-
dose, another life wasted. I arrived, parked on the roof as usual and
headed into the Trauma Intensive Care Unit (ICU). I introduced myself to
the nurse, the resident and the cardiology fellow on his ICU rotation. The
patient was a 35-year-old Hispanic male, brought in after a drug overdose,
prescription drugs as usual. Nobody dies from heroin overdoses anymore,
everyone takes the wrong combination of prescription medications and
then adds a little alcohol and it's over. The patient seemed like a typical
inner-city hoodlum — many tattoos, scars from fights or shootings. Reli-
gious medallions hung around the bed and a large Hispanic family was
in the waiting room, possibly his but who knows. I did my initial assessment. The patient seemed healthy other than his drug problem; the labs all
seemed OK. He wasn't brain dead, not yet anyway, but had a fluid collection pressing on his brain, which had been lacking adequate oxygen supply
for an undetermined amount of time. His kidneys, being the first organs the
body sacrifices for survival, were functioning fine so he wasn't down too
long. Lab values for creatinine or kidney function can give us an estimate
of how long a person was unresponsive before being found. This is called
acute renal failure and is usually reversible. He was donor designated so
upon arrival in the ICU I checked to see if he had taken any blood products over the last 48 hours, filled out the appropriate form with the blood
plasma volume calculations and requested the nurse draw off our blood

samples and send them for infectious disease testing. I ran through his lab reports since he was admitted and filled out as much of our own chart as possible. I logged into my laptop and updated the active patient system to document what reflexes he had left, what the status with the family was and whether he had any issues that the next Transplant Coordinator (TC) would need to know. I touched base with the nurse and the fellow, told them we would be following the patient by phone for now and to please call us if anything changed.

Typical of patients who were not brain dead, we monitored this patient's condition for over a week by phone. I kept an eye on the case notes and saw that a TC had spoken with his family and obtained consent. His family had decided to wait and see if he progressed over the next 72 hours but had decided that they would withdraw life support by turning off the ventilator if he did not progress to brain death. The TC who obtained consent from the family explained to them the process for donation called "Donation after Cardiac Death" or DCD as we called it. DCD was actually the way organ donation started, before Harvard created the brain death criteria. These donors are not brain dead, they are irreversibly brain injured, the majority of the time to a severe degree. There is a much smaller window of opportunity for donation in the case of DCD. The patients can only be between about three and 45 years old. They can only donate the liver and kidneys because the patient is extubated or taken off the ventilator in the Operating Room (OR) and sedated. Only brain-dead donors can donate heart, lungs or pancreas. They have to die within 60 to 90 minutes because the organs can't handle more time without appropriate blood flow or oxygen. Some Organ Procurement Organizations (OPO's) actually cannulate, or place large-bore tubings that help flush the organs into the donor's femoral arteries. This makes it possible to immediately infuse preservation fluids. Thankfully, we did not have to do this. Once my next on-call rotation came up I knew I was headed there because I had already been involved with the case.

I arrived in the morning. It was a sunny fall day, crisp air up on the roof of the garage. I saw some great cityscapes while I was on all those hospital roofs. I packed my bag with everything I would need from supplies kept in my trunk. It looked as if the family was coming in to talk to me according to the notes from the night before. As I got off the elevator some family members were starting to arrive and I heard them saying I was the "organ donor lady" as I walked past. I went into the ICU and spoke again with the fellow and nurse who had been with me last week. They updated me on what was happening. The patient was relatively stable except for having some issues with his blood pressure, which was not unusual for donors. The kidneys and liver were doing fine, the labs were all normal, the infectious disease results were back and the patient did not have Hepatitis B or C, HIV and no infections were brewing. Things looked good.

The ICU staff at first believed he may have stopped overbreathing the ventilator that morning. Overbreathing was the term we used to describe what happened when a patient took extra breaths in addition to what the ventilator was already providing. Overbreathing was usually the last reflex to go because the brain stem is responsible for breathing and heart rate. The neurosurgeon was expected any minute to start the brain death exams. As I was updating my Administrator on Call (AOC), the neurology team arrived. I overheard the attending physician from the neurology service who had come to assess if the patient was brain dead make a comment that made me uncomfortable, something like, "let's get this over with, this has gone on long enough." They went into the patient's room and closed the door and curtain, which made me more uncomfortable still. I hung up and walked into the room, introduced myself as the TC and asked if I could watch. They didn't seem very happy about it but it was all part of the process and they knew it. There were no pupils, no corneals, no cough or gag, no withdraw to painful stimuli and the patient tested positive for doll's eyes. Then the cold calorics. One of the residents held the patient's eyelids open and they squirted 30 cc of ice-cold fluid into his left ear canal. I was standing at the foot of the bed looking straight at him, they squirted 30 cc in the right ear and we all watched as his eyes slowly but surely drifted downward to his right side. That was the first and only time in two and a half years that I saw a reaction to cold calorics, but there was no doubt in my mind I saw it. The attending neurologist said something about coming to do second exam in 12 hours until I said, "wait a minute, his eyes moved." One doctor stormed out of the room and the neurology fellow stayed, but he too agreed — his eyes had moved. The patient was not brain dead; I said I would go and speak to the family about DCD.

The TC who worked the case before me had done a great job with the family, they were prepared, asked appropriate questions and had all gathered to be part of the decision. There were about 30 people present, some of whom did not speak English. They told me that the donor's 15-year-old daughter was on her way to say her goodbyes so I took the opportunity to do what we called a respiratory drive assessment. This is a test where we attempt to mimic how the patient will do once extubated. We basically disconnect the patient from the ventilator but do not pull out the breathing tube and then watch his vital signs, some change right away, some change initially then are stable for an hour at times. Some families like to be present for this test and I felt it was helpful to them in understanding what would happen when the patient would be extubated. When we are in the process of dying the first thing that happens is that our heart rate, blood pressure and respiratory rate increase in an effort to save the brain while the oxygen saturation, which should be around 98 percent to 100 percent, drops. But if the oxygen saturation or amount of oxygen in the blood drops to 80 percent or less on a person who does not have Chronic Obstructive Pulmonary Disorder (COPD) such as asthma or emphysema, we stop and reconnect the ventilator. Patients who have any kind of COPD are pretty much used to struggling for air so they can sometimes go for hours or a day without the ventilator, but with an oxygen saturation below 80 percent, before their heart stops. These patients are not DCD candidates, we need to be reasonably sure the patient's heart will stop within 60 to 90 minutes. This patient was very close to brain death, so most of his brain was not functioning and his vital signs changed within minutes. I checked with his family and his daughter had arrived so I went to get the cardiology fellow to help with the final discussion.

We all gathered in a small room. It was hot and people were sitting in chairs, on the floor and tables and some are standing. When we came in they closed the door and opened a spot against the wall for us. They were grieving but most seemed to have already found closure and were ready to let him go. He had struggled for many years with his drug addictions but he was still their little brother — the youngest of seven — four sisters and three brothers, all of them there. The doctor started by saying how sorry he was that they couldn't save him. He said, "I'm sorry he has to die" and got choked up. The next thing I knew he was crying and trying to talk between sobs, then he quickly excused himself from the room leaving me alone with the family. Pretty much everyone was crying, I started to say something about how hard the doctors had tried to save the man's life and how involved they had become, as they had just witnessed.

We discussed some of the details of the actual DCD, where it would take place, what would happen after and when they would know the outcome. Then his oldest sister said, "I just don't want him to die alone," and they all nodded their heads in agreement. I looked her right in the eyes and said, "I promise he will not die alone. I promise I will be with him the entire time. I will not leave his side. I will treat him as if he were my brother." They said they trusted me and believed that I would keep my word. Then, one-by-one, they filed out of the room to go say their final goodbye to their brother.

I tried to focus on allocating the liver but it was extremely difficult with all that was going on in front of me. They were praying and crying, some of the men showing anger, some needing to kneel down on the floor as they comforted each other. Then his daughter went in and they asked me to come into the room and began to show me pictures from an old album his daughter had brought of him holding her on his lap when she was little. They wanted me to see that he was more than just another drug addict, more than this lifeless person laying here in the ICU. He was a person and he was loved by many. They said their goodbyes, thanked me and the staff on the way out and made sure I had all their phone numbers to call after the OR procedures were done.

I had placed the liver quickly with a young Hispanic male who was in the same hospital, although we were not allowed to tell anything about the race of a recipient to the donor family. The kidneys were going back to my office to be "pumped," which improves the function of the donor kidneys outside of the donor, requiring them to be pumped with cold preservation fluid for as long as 48 hours before transplanting.

I spoke with the charge nurse in the OR, she was someone I had worked with before and liked very much so I was relieved it was her on duty. She immediately became my friend one night when in the middle of a long case she brought me a hot, fresh cup of coffee to sneak into the substerile room outside the OR. We didn't need anesthesia for DCD's and the ICU staff was ready to go. The recovering surgeons were from the same hospital so setting an OR time was pretty quick and easy. So we packed everything up and headed down to the OR together.

We got into the OR, talked to the surgeon, reviewed the necessary paperwork and they got into their scrubs and begin to prep and drape the patient. The surgeons always leave the room during extubation and do not return until five minutes after pronouncement. The pronouncing doctor remains to pronounce the patient dead. During prepping one surgeon pulled the cardiac leads off the patient's chest and made a comment that it looked like a "herpes outbreak" underneath one of the leads. I strongly disagreed and said it looked like a whitehead, a pimple, nothing to be worried about. I reminded him we had reviewed all the patient's past medical history and serology testing. They left the room and the resident from the ICU who came in with us cut the air cuff tube on the endotracheal tube and slid the tube out of the patient's mouth. The ICU nurse had already started pushing morphine into the IV so he didn't struggle.

I sat at one side of the head of the bed, quietly recording the vital signs minute by minute as his life began to slip away. The OR staff were silent. There was only the beeping of the monitor. I noticed after a few minutes that the patient has started to perspire on his forehead and appeared to be struggling to breathe. His body was shutting down as he was unable to get enough oxygen into his bloodstream to survive. The nurse gave more morphine; we stayed completely separated from that process because we never ever wanted to create the perception that the TC's had hastened death to get at the organs quicker. I watched as he continued to perspire and tense the muscles in his forehead. I went over to him and pulled my stool up close to the head of the bed and began to gently stroke his forehead. As I had promised his siblings, I assured him he was not alone and that it was OK to let go. I just kept quietly saying in his ear that he could go when he was ready until finally we no longer heard the monitor and he was no longer struggling. The resident slipped his stethoscope into a sterile sleeve and the surgical tech moved it into place over the heart, he looked at his watch and said, "time of death, 3:38 a.m." Then he signed the paperwork and solemnly walked out. I thanked him on his way out, thanked the ICU nurse for her help and turned to let the surgeons in at exactly the five-minute mark.

The surgeons made the incision and got immediately to the aorta, cannulating with the tubing for the preservation fluid, dumping basins of sterile ice into the abdomen. Today, OR's have sterile ice machine makers, but I recall when I worked in the OR a long time ago that we had to send the organ donor team up to the cafeteria to get buckets of ice. The perfusionists from the OPO also bring frozen bags of sterile fluid that they break up with big hammers on the back table. It doesn't take long to get the liver out. It looked good but the first surgeon had told the attending surgeon about the alleged herpes, so he told me he was declining the liver for his patient. I alerted my AOC, who was not happy. I immediately called the first backup surgeon on my list, he asked which surgeon was with me and, when I told him, it turned out they knew each other, so he said, "Let me talk to him." I held the phone up to the surgeon's ear as his hands were still inside the patient and he proceeded to tell the backup surgeon that the donor had what appeared to be herpes! I snatched the phone away and told the surgeon on the phone that was incorrect, they were wrong, and asked for them to give me a chance to prove it. I promised to call him back. My AOC instructed me to get an Emergency Room (ER) doctor to come up and take a look. I have no idea how I managed to talk an ER doctor into coming up to the OR at 4 a.m. to look at what I swore was a whitehead, but somehow I did. I'm sure I sounded as desperate as I felt.

I was flaming pissed because the liver was about to be wasted and for no reason. The ER doctor came in, uncovered the chest, looked at the lesion in question and said, "Looks like a whitehead to me. From the lead adhesive probably." I wanted to cry. I had the surgeon paged through the intercom and when he came back, the ER doctor told him what he thought. The surgeon looked at me and said he was very sorry. Of course, by now the liver was no good.

The donor did save two lives that night, two people's lives changed forever because of him. I remained in contact with his sister for about a year. She said they would never forget me, but I knew it was the other way around, I would never forget her or her family.

■

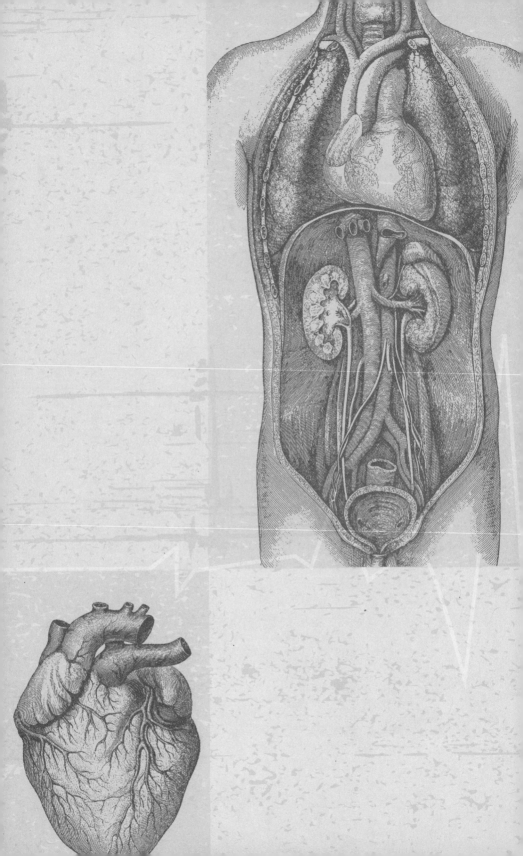

6

A Typical Day on Call

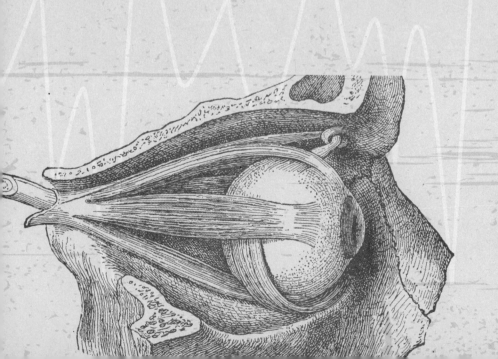

ONE DAY I WAS ON MY WAY TO AN INNER-CITY HOSPITAL WHERE THE donor was listed as a "Jane Doe," meant to indicate of course that her identity was unknown. These cases are really hard to handle. If you can't locate next of kin you can't move forward, so we would go to exhaustive lengths to find family members. I arrived on the unit and introduced myself to the nurse who signed me into the computer system so I could update my lab results. Another Transplant Coordinator had started things the day before with the initial referral. I sat down at the desk to familiarize myself with the details of this case. Female, probably over 300 pounds, approximately 30-years-old, Jane Doe, was in a motor vehicle accident with a man. She was the passenger, the male was taken to another hospital and was in critical condition. This patient had a small piece of folded toilet paper in her pants pocket with a phone number written on it. I walked into the room to take a look at her IV's and how her blood pressure was holding up.

She had massive abdominal injuries and had been taken immediately to the Operating Room (OR) with the trauma team. Like many patients in motor vehicle accidents, her intestines were swollen to the point that her abdomen could not be closed after the incision. Hospitals do different things in this situation, but a common way and the one they had used that time was to cut open IV bags so they were like sheets of thick plastic and sew them into the abdominal wall. The bags act as a covering to the intestines but allow for swelling and quick access if necessary. As the swelling goes down and the patient becomes more stable they eventually go back to the OR and close the abdomen. She was stable at that point.

I called my Administrator on Call (AOC) to fill him in on what was happening and he asked if they had identified her yet. "No, not yet" I told him, "but I will get working on it." After reviewing the notes from the previous TC I paged the on-call public relations person, it was a Sunday. She called back in about five minutes and as soon as I said I was from the Organ Donor Program she lit into me. She was yelling and rambling on about not telling her what to do, she had done her job for a long time and identified many Jane Does. I attempted a few times to interrupt her but was unsuccessful. She was really worked up — the problem was, I wasn't the TC who got her that way. So I let her just vent until she was done and then I politely explained to her that we had never spoken before and this was my first time on this case. Of course she started apologizing like crazy and explained to me that the TC the day before had been screaming at her on the phone that people's lives were at risk if she didn't come in and have the patient's picture shown on the news. The public relations director did not feel it was appropriate to show a picture of a critically ill patient in her condition at this point.

The nurses told me they called the phone number on the piece of toilet paper and it was a male who definitely did not want to be called again. This whole situation was looking very suspicious. While I was there we got word from the other hospital that the male driver of the car had died and his wife was at the hospital with him. I'm pretty sure whatever they were doing together wasn't good. The accident happened late on a Friday night in a very bad section of town.

As I was updating our computer database on my laptop an instructor from one of the local nursing programs approached me and asked if I would mind explaining to her students what we did. I told her I would be glad to and about 12 adult nursing students gathered around me. As I was explaining to them how we evaluate donors I heard the monitors in the patient's room sound an alarm. Suddenly there were lots of people heading toward her room. Residents, other nurses and someone with the unit crash cart. She was getting ready to code and go into cardiac arrest. The trauma director was a small, highly respected female. She had very short, spiky hair and was attractive, but oddly always had on a perfectly clean pair of Timberland boots. Dressed in scrubs or street clothes, it didn't matter. She started to give orders for medication and Advanced Cardiac Life Support (ACLS). Basically ACLS is an algorithm for what drugs to give, when to give them and how much to give. The drugs are always given in the same order. Drugs like Atropine and Epinephrine will kick start the heart. She looked at me and asked what my plan was. Since the woman was still a Jane Doe I didn't really have a plan. We made the decision to start chest compressions while I made a couple last-ditch phone calls. I gathered up the nursing class students and told them to round robin with compressions until I told them to stop. Most needed stools to stand on because the woman was very large. It was a total mess because every time someone compressed her chest, fluids leaked out of her open abdomen. I headed out to the hallway and called my AOC to let him know the situation was looking bad. I told him about the public relations person and my interactions with her, and then I reviewed what we knew about the man with her in the car. She was with a man who was married to someone else, she has no identification at all on her except the phone number on the toilet paper, a phone number of someone who didn't want to talk to us. The area where the accident occurred was a highly active prostitution section. I couldn't believe my AOC was still silent on the other end of the phone. "Hello?" I said. He made a noise and said he was thinking. I walked toward the room again and they were still at it, student after student doing chest compressions keeping her organs perfused with oxygen and blood. Finally, I couldn't stand the waiting any longer and said, "Can't you see, she's a prostitute? That would be a huge risk." He agreed and allowed me to call off the code. What a shame. I hope they found her family; no one should die nameless. She was surely someone's sister, aunt, daughter, mother or friend.

Typically, during a 24- to 48-hour shift I would be going from hospital to hospital evaluating people in various stages of death or critical illness. I have seen people with horrific head injuries and some of the craziest stuff you could ever imagine. One man had a sinus infection that he let go too long without treatment and it literally ate a hole through his sinus cavity and right into his brain. I've seen patients with fungal infections to the brain that were so serious you could clearly see where it was eating away the brain tissue by the random black holes on a CT scan. It was not uncommon while being on a unit doing an evaluation that word would travel around the hospital that the TC was there and suddenly you would have four referrals to follow up on. I feel that this running around is what burns most of us out. It really is nothing but tragedy and death. Even though I've written about cases where there were lives saved and families comforted, the cases that went nowhere for various reasons far outweigh the good. Sometimes, after many hours of work, things just fell apart. We had to do things to follow through sometimes that were emotionally painful for us.

I was assigned to a case once where the patient was a foreign sailor who had fallen off the top deck of the ship onto the lowest deck and suffered a massive closed-head injury. I arrived at the hospital and went to an area that the TC's affectionately called the "Monkey Cage." It was a small, glass-enclosed corner of the unit that had a counter, some equipment and computers. It was where the staff wanted us to sit. We had to talk to the employer of the sailor first who helped us figure out where the sailor was from and if he had any family back home. He was from an island somewhere near the Philippines.

There are so many challenges in dealing with other cultures. Many cultures have beliefs and rituals surrounding the dying process that were at times impossible to overcome. In this situation I had no idea what to expect but my AOC insisted that I be on the phone when the physician told the patient's wife that her husband had died. We calculated the time difference and although it was late at night at our location it was around 3 p.m. in the Philippines. So with everyone on a three-way call we dialed the number and a female voice answered the phone. The interpreter explained that he was with an American doctor who needed to speak to her. The doctor began speaking, taking breaks so the interpreter could translate what the doctor was saying into her language. He told her that her husband had suffered a very serious accident and that his brain was injured beyond what they could fix. Finally he said that he was very sorry but her husband was dead. She started screaming on the other end of the phone, literally wailing in emotional pain. The doctor and I were both crying because, despite the language barrier, the sound of grief and pain is universal.

We had no idea if she had someone there with her when suddenly the line went dead. It is hard for me to describe how it felt sitting there, thinking about how she must have felt. She couldn't understand us, couldn't get to her husband, we didn't even know that she fully understood what we told her. We called back but the phone just rang and rang. We called the employer back and explained what happened and finally got a number for another next of kin listed in his file. We did not even know how this person was related to the sailor but we had no choice but to call. So with everyone back on the phone we did the whole thing again and the person turned out to be the patient's sister. We explained what had happened, that her brother was mortally injured in a ship accident and her sister-in-law had gotten hysterical, hung up and would not answer our calls. This was not going to work out for us at all. I had one minute or less to ask about organ donation. The interpreter tried to explain that many Americans who die of brain injuries donate their organs to people who are living but very ill. The sister said she did not understand what we were talking about and I gave up. This one was just too challenging to overcome. I will never forget the sound of her crying though, never.

Cultural differences played a part in a very interesting experience I had with a Vietnamese family at an inner-city hospital. I was still in training so I was sent to be with a senior TC. When I first arrived on the unit there were many family members in the room with the patient. Most of them were women. The TC brought me up to date on what was happening. The man had had a massive stroke two days earlier and appeared to be brain dead. His wife, daughter and her fiancé were with the patient. According to their customs, if her father died before she was married she would need to wait for a period of one year from his death to get married. It was May and their wedding, which they had been working on for over a year, was planned for June. So the hospital agreed to wait before making a brain death pronouncement until a Buddhist monk could come and marry the couple right there in the room. Fortunately, at this hospital it was easy to find a Buddhist monk since it served a very large Buddhist community. It took about an hour to pull everything together, but the daughter was married in the hospital room with her father present at her side. The family said they would still have the ceremony in June but now we were free to pronounce him and speak to the family. The brain death pronouncement didn't take very long because they had been preparing in the background while the wedding ceremony was taking place. The daughter and son-in-law were translating for the doctors and nurses. Once we knew they all understood the father was dead despite being on the ventilator we entered the room and introduced ourselves to the man's daughter and wife. The daughter was doing her best to explain to her mother what we were asking and I was not really optimistic this was going to work out.

The TC asked if any family members had or needed a kidney transplant — aha — the magic words. They started talking very quickly to one another again and the daughter remained quiet while the ladies talked.

Then, all of sudden the daughter said that her aunts claimed one of their sisters had a kidney transplant five years ago and was still alive because of it. They could not speak English and we really didn't know what the daughter was telling them, which is the main reason we usually do not allow family to translate, but it didn't matter. They understood that a family in this exact situation had said yes to donation and that it had saved their sister's life, so they would help someone else and also say yes.

At that same hospital I had another very difficult family situation with an inner-city African American family. The patient was a 52-year-old male who suffered a severe bleed into his brain. He collapsed getting off the bus right outside the hospital, some of his family believed he didn't feel well and was coming to the Emergency Room (ER). Unfortunately he came just a little too late. It appeared he could be a full donor and I was moving ahead with the preparations for that. The staff had done the first brain death exam and had informed the family but had chosen to wait 24 hours before second exam as he was stable. Then the challenges began — the woman claiming to be his legal wife was not his wife according to some of his children. Some of the adult children were his and some were hers. One of the physicians had aggravated the situation by insisting on seeing a marriage certificate before speaking to her. The man had been there less than 12 hours and the wife had already been removed twice already by security for screaming at the staff. I always felt she was lucky that she was in that hospital; they were a tough group and allowed for families to do many things other hospitals would not allow. One of the nurses on the unit felt it was perfect that I was the TC onsite. She felt I would handle the woman better than most. "Is that a compliment?" I asked, and we all cracked up. Just then, she arrived. The wife who was kicked out less than three hours earlier was back with one of the craziest wigs I had ever seen on her head. To complicate matters I got the results of our serology testing back from the office and he was classified as "HCV NAT +" or, in other words, actively infected with Hepatitis C.

There go the heart and lungs. No positive serology thoracic organs were transplanted except in the very rare instance of a positive recipient, but that would be with inactive or past infections, not recent ones. So, to complicate the relations between the family and staff, the attending physician was now required by law to inform the wife her husband had an active Hepatitis C infection and she would need to get tested herself. Not surprisingly the doctor was very unhappy he had to do this.

Many times people think the hospital staff welcome the TC's presence and like taking part in the process but that couldn't be further from the truth. Some of them despised seeing us on the unit, both nurses and doctors. For a nurse it meant the busiest shift you could have aside from multiple codes. There are central lines to be placed, hundreds of labs to be drawn every four hours, exact monitoring of intake and output, blood to be given that has to be double checked by two Registered Nurses before starting each unit, bedside tests like echocardiograms and bronchoscopies to be done plus dealing with the family and the TC's who could be extremely pushy. I remember one nurse telling me she should put on her roller skates when we were there.

When it was my turn to talk to the wife and children I took them to a small conference room that doubled as our nap quarters whenever we were lucky enough to get a 15-minute nap in a 28-hour case. We sat around a table and as soon as I started asking if they understood what was happening the arguing started. I didn't even know what the hell they were all fighting about, yelling at each other, obviously angry over what had happened. I was in a closed room with three angry males and two women all virtually out of control. I thought to myself, shit, I have already broken the number one rule from working in psych — never put them between yourself and the door. I loudly said, "Do you know that the vast majority of the 6,000 people in this city waiting for kidneys are African Americans?" They were silent. They were all staring at me. The patient's wife said, "Get the paperwork and

I will sign it." The patient saved two lives with the donation of his kidneys to recipients who were Hepatitis C positive and would otherwise not have received an organ.

That was what it was like to be on call. There were many times that you went in, started the paperwork, sent off serology tests to our lab and instructed the staff by calling three times a day to ask about medications, reflexes, problems and family issues. Some days you wanted to flush your pager down the toilet, toss it off a bridge or out the car window. When the pager gods were quiet all of us watched the computer board knowing exactly who would be going out next. The worst was if you had been out all day the first call day and you get home exhausted, you eat anything that is easy, get in bed and just as you lay your head down the pager goes off. These were the times I would literally need to cry for five minutes and feel sorry for myself before calling the Clinical Phone Coordinator and Administrator on Call to find out where I was going. Then you reminded yourself as you listened to the details, at least the patient being evaluated isn't me or anyone in my family. You get dressed again and hit the road.

■

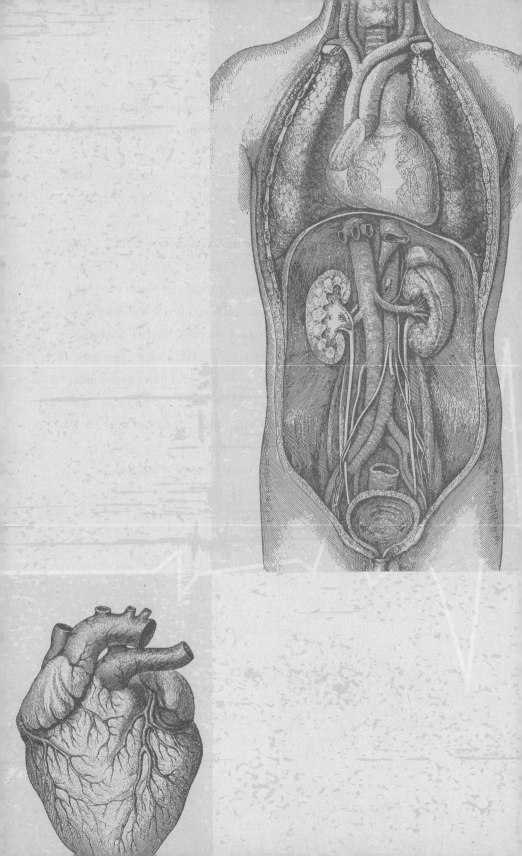

7

It's Like the Wild, Wild West

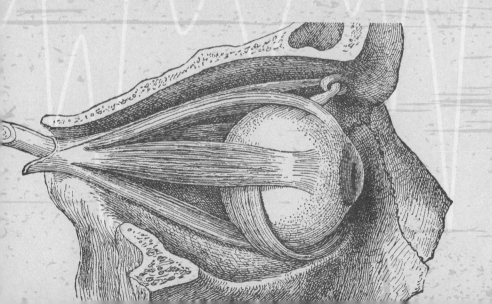

I WENT TO SO MANY SHOOTINGS I LOST COUNT BUT THERE ARE A FEW THAT still to this day stand out for me and I'll never forget. When your pager goes off in the middle of the night there is an 80 percent chance it will be a case involving a shooting, especially on the weekends. On this occasion, I jumped in the shower more to wake myself up than to get clean; clean hair meant nothing when someone was dying. I headed out the door and called the number I was given by the Clinical Phone Coordinator (CPC). The patient was still in the Trauma Bay, never a good sign. I called and asked for the person who called in the referral, it was the chief trauma resident at a huge inner-city hospital. He told me the patient was bleeding out, "he transected his internal carotid artery, I could pour the whole blood bank in this kid and it won't matter." I reminded him the patient had organ donor designation on his license and that he should do everything reasonably possible to keep him going until I could get there in about 45 minutes. He said he would do what he could, but no promises. I called and updated my Administrator on Call and he said right away that I should have pushed him to keep giving blood. Oh man, I thought, this was not going to be good.

I arrived at the hospital and headed down to the Trauma Bay on the street level. As I walked through the doors there were many hysterical crying people outside, they could have been for my guy, although you never knew. I did notice two very pregnant women both visibly upset. I got to the

Trauma Bay itself and it looked like a war zone. It was one big room with multiple areas to work on people, but there was blood and trash all over the place and cops everywhere. Finally I made contact with my resident and he told me this kid had been practically without a blood pressure for over two hours and his kidneys were probably junk. As I called my AOC to give him an update, the trauma team started chest compressions on the patient. I made a couple of rapid phone calls to the office and the lab and as I was talking the resident brought in the family to see him before he died. Included in this group were both pregnant women I had seen outside, both totally hysterical, screaming and crying. It is so hard to watch scenes like this unfold. I have watched them again and again in this job and it never gets any easier. The resident escorted the family back out and walked up to me and said, "Are you planning on doing a rapid recovery on this kid, because if you are I am going to need to call in some help. He is our 12th shooting this shift and we are spent." I told him that would be up to the family and I needed to speak with them. The hospital chaplain showed up and we walked together outside onto the sidewalk. We didn't see anyone but a homeless guy and a security guard. I asked the guard where the patient's family went and he told me, "Labor and delivery, both ladies were having labor pains." Oh no. I knew there was no way out of this, I had to talk to that family. This was a 21-year-old and my organization would not be happy to lose his kidneys and liver.

What we called a rapid recovery was only done in extreme situations. It happened when the donor became so unstable he could not be kept going. We talked to the family very quickly in those cases and if they wanted to move forward we asked the attending to pronounce and then we would resume chest compressions (not CPR) until a surgeon arrived. As an organization we had been known to do compressions for over two hours just to get a liver and a couple kidneys. That was when you rounded up every medical and nursing student in the hospital to take turns doing compressions — it was vital the blood be kept circulating. The problem was, you had to present the family with this option quickly and it was not easy for them to understand how we could keep someone going to get their organs but not to save their life.

I gave a quick call to my AOC who, as I predicted, directed me to find the family. The chaplain and I walked up to the labor and delivery floor, which typical of city hospitals seemed like four city blocks away! The chaplain left me out by the elevators and went to find them, saying she would be back for me. I must have stood there for about 10 minutes and it was possibly the longest 10 minutes of my life. Finally, after what seemed like an eternity, she came out to get me and we went back into a small room where the patient's parents were sitting. Both the patient's mother and sister were more than eight months pregnant and the stress was causing them to have contractions. I got right to the point, I was from the organ donor program and I was there because their son had chosen to be an organ donor on his license and unfortunately we were at the point that a decision had to be made fast. I apologized for having to approach them so abruptly but if we didn't act quickly the opportunity would be lost. They looked at each other, you could tell this was just horrifying for them, but they wholeheartedly agreed that we should do whatever we could to fulfill his wish. I asked them to please not go anywhere because I would need them to sign paperwork while we got a surgeon there. I headed as fast as I could back down to the Trauma Bay. I walked in and the nurses were holding a Doppler (an ultrasound that records blood flow over a patient's chest). I started to say, "Good news, they want to … oh no, he has no heartbeat?" Great. I updated my AOC and he was not happy; they had only given the patient 19 units of blood, he felt they could have given much more and as one of our biggest transplant hospitals they were expected to go above and beyond the norm to make donation happen. My AOC told me to obtain consent from them for tissue donation.

Tissue donation is something very different from organ donation. After the first time I saw a tissue recovery in the Operating Room (OR) when I was still a surgical tech I felt it was necessary, but something no one should ever have to witness. Once a patient was already dead the tissue team would come in. While we could transplant organs from donors with Hepatitis C or B, we couldn't donate tissue if you had any positive serology results. Tissue donation is Food and Drug Administration (FDA) regulated and every single operating room in the country has a closet full of various kinds of dried bone graft and most have other things in the freezers. When I worked in the OR we had bone cubes, bone screws (literally screws made out of cadaver bone), bone struts that were rectangular shaped and bone matrix that would allow and encourage bone to grow where there is a deficit. We also had a freezer in the pathology lab that held the patellar tendons used for ACL repairs and we had a frozen femoral head for a while that one surgeon thought he would need and didn't use. These things were all regulated just like any implant they put in your body. The tissue processors could turn a donor down if they had multiple tattoos, had served time in prison or if they answered "yes" to any of the following questions: did the donor ever have sex in exchange for money or drugs? Did the donor ever engage in sexual activity with another male (if the donor is male). On the positive side, one tissue donor can enhance the lives of up to 50 people.

The tissue team, who are usually either surgical techs, OR nurses or even a few surgeons from foreign countries, take your femurs (long thigh bones), humerus (long bone in the upper arm), tibias (larger bone in the lower leg), patellar tendons, Achilles tendons and the quadriceps tendon. Then they take skin, usually from the back, and if corneas were consented as well, the eye bank comes to get the corneas. I always felt that corneal donation was kind of underestimated and encouraged families to at least consent to that, it can even be done in the morgue. If the heart isn't donated they can use it for valves. They literally hold the heart in their hand and cut through the wall with scissors, and then they cut out the aortic and mitral valves. They also recover saphenous veins from the legs and this Organ Procurement Organization (OPO) actually held the record for recovering the longest vein intact in the country.

I went back to the family and sat with the parents, most likely younger than myself, and we went through the patient's medical and social history. The form consisted of 20 pages of questions about everything you could ask medically but many of the questions, if answered yes, put you in a high-risk category for HIV and they would decline the donation. As I asked if the patient had ever been hospitalized they told me that this was his third shooting in six months. I couldn't believe it, I'd spent the last six hours on this case and they would definitely turn him down as a donor. I only hoped the eye bank would take and use his corneas. I wanted to give something to this grieving family. His corneas were donated — they were young, healthy, clear corneas and someone is hopefully looking through them right now.

In another case the shooting was self-inflicted. A kid walked into the bar where his girlfriend of three months worked and shot himself in the chin. Chaos, of course, and he was brought into the nearest trauma center and we were called. As I got to the unit I found the nurses working furiously on this kid. This hospital has rather close quarters and the nurses' station desk is only about 10 feet from the patient's room. The nurses can't find his parents, he is not donor designated and he is grossly unstable. The girlfriend was in the room and her mother arrived, they went into the hall to talk and the girl kept saying she didn't know why he did it. The nurses were busy working on him so I approached the girlfriend and asked her if she knew where his parents were. She said they had only been living together for three months in an apartment and she didn't know where the parents lived. I make a few quick phone calls, to my AOC, of course, letting him know I was in a potential rapid recovery situation, which prompted him to make calls getting perfusion moving and another TC headed toward me. I called our office because they were frantically searching the internet for his parents; they would use sites like Intelius and had credit cards for paid searches. I was trying to fax lab results to the office so they could start looking for liver and kidney recipients. I had to call the medical examiner's office and let them know I was on site. The donor was not dead but very unstable so I knew they wanted him. The investigator from the medical examiner's office asked me, "What are you looking to take?" I told the investigator just liver and kidneys, if they were any good after this, and he gave me the OK. I told him I would call him when we were done in the OR and they could come get him. Just as I hung up I saw the patient's blood pressure dropping, from 90/60 to 70/50 — shit, he was going to code. All the residents ran in the room, one stopped to ask me what they should use for his blood pressure. I told him the drug we preferred because it didn't hurt the kidneys and how much to give. I also told him to get the fluids wide open, something we did when a patient was crashing that allowed the IV fluids to flow into the patient at a greater rate than the IV pumps delivered, which helped stabilize blood pressure. Then, thank god, I saw my coworker running into the unit. She saw what was going on and called the OR first to let them know we may have had a rapid recovery and started getting a kidney or liver surgeon paged immediately. I changed into scrubs and thought, damn it, this is what you try so hard to avoid having to do, but I had no choice.

When I came out of the bathroom, they were in the middle of a full code. The trauma director had arrived and he and his team were working as hard as they could. The girlfriend was getting hysterical watching them do chest compressions. The trauma doctor walked up and told me he couldn't keep him going any longer, he needed to call it, a term frequently used to call off a code or stop trying to save the patient. I looked at him and said, "OK, well if you can pronounce him we will restart compressions until the surgeon can get here." He said, "You want me to do what? So you can do what?" Of course there were at least three expletives in those questions as well. I got my AOC on the phone and told him what was happening and he asked to speak to the trauma doctor.

There was total bedlam at this point as one of the patients in a room across from the desk became agitated and tried to get out of his room. The hall was packed with people including the OR charge nurse and the on-call anesthesiologist. As the trauma doctor hung up the phone with my boss, the nurses pushed his bed into the hall with one nurse sitting on top of him doing compressions. I will never forget what she said to me — "Someone's going to get this heart tonight!" — as she pumped away. I didn't want to tell her we couldn't take his heart like that. They pronounced him and restarted compressions as we had asked, my coworker was talking to the girlfriend again but she really had no idea what to do. This was all going on in a space so narrow that only one person could be alongside the bed at a time. Thankfully, one of the kidney surgeons showed up and was the voice of reason. He stated we could not get his kidneys placed without a medical and social history. Without the patient's parents we didn't have that so he suggested we stop. I checked in with AOC and just as quickly as it had all started, I told the team to stop compressions. He was gone. A totally wasted life, leaving devastation in the aftermath, all because of a single, irrational, bad decision. But it was amazing to watch the trauma team desperately trying to preserve the organs for donation.

Another potential donor we worked on actually survived in the end. A young man had gotten into an argument with another guy on his street over a parking spot and pulled his gun to be a show off. What he didn't realize was that the man was an off-duty city cop and he was trained to react when someone pointed a gun at him. It wasn't clear who shot first but the kid ended up with his liver practically split into two pieces by the bullet.

It was still dark when I pulled into a spot on the roof of the parking garage. As I headed toward the Emergency Room entrance I saw people everywhere, crying, yelling and praying. I checked in with the security officer and he decided to escort me up to the Intensive Care Unit (ICU). We walked through halls lined with people there for that kid. His family was in the ICU waiting room so the guard took me through a back door to the ICU to avoid the family. They had both big glass doors open and there were people in there. There were six bags of blood hanging at once on something called a rapid infuser. I headed to the desk, grabbed the chart and got to work. I knew that if he coded I was going to have to talk to the family and there were so many people I really didn't want to be the one to approach them. The trauma surgeon stopped by and told me he did everything he could, the patient's liver was packed with multiple sponges to try and stop the profuse bleeding but the blood was going out as fast as it was coming in. The surgeon had put the patient under some deep sedation to keep him from fighting but from what he could tell the kid still had reflexes. He said he was going to get some sleep and told the nurses to page him if the kid got worse. This was truly the most incredible example of trauma nursing at its best.

In these extreme situations patients are given huge amounts of blood. They are first given blood that matches their blood type, but if they receive what's called uncrossmatched blood, that's a sign things are really bad. It also made life more difficult on us since we had to account for all the blood given. Not just packed red cells, but also fresh frozen plasma, which is given many times when patients are bleeding liters and liters of fluids. As part of the serology testing we had to calculate how much blood in the samples was the patient's and how much blood was from the blood donor. We performed a calculation based on how much the patient weighed multiplied by the amount of blood and fluids given over the last 48 hours to determine if we were really testing the patient's blood or the blood bank's blood. In this case he had gotten more blood than I had ever seen so we called the hospital lab and asked for samples of the blood that had been taken when the patient was admitted and before any transfusions had been given.

My AOC wanted me to contact the medical examiner to get approval for donation in case the patient turned into a rapid recovery. I did attempt to talk with the AOC several times, saying that the whole reason we did compressions was to circulate blood but if this kid codes it's because he has exsanguinated or bled out. She didn't care about that. So I called the medical examiner's office and spoke with one of the regular investigators. She immediately said she wasn't sure if they would allow us to take his kidneys because he had been shot by a cop, possibly because of the legal implications, and they had very few details. She said she would check with the on-call pathologist and call me back. I waited, watching the family who were shocked and devastated. I remember the father had on overalls and I knew he wasn't from the inner city. I have seen some impressive lifesaving efforts but this case was by far the most impressive. The nurses were literally running for supplies. Blood needed to be checked by two Registered Nurses (RN's) before it could be hung and these girls were hanging four or five bags at a time. The room looked as if there had been a massacre.

My Blackberry rang and it was the investigator from the medical examiner's office. She said she was sorry, they almost always were supportive of donations, but this time the pathologist on call said no way. Because of the police's involvement and the lack of information surrounding the incident, they were not comfortable allowing the donation. I completely understood but said that, unfortunately, I was sure she would hear back from me. Of course my AOC said that was not acceptable and to call them back and find out exactly what more information they needed and find a way to get them answers.

Oh OK, I thought to myself, no problem. How the hell was I going to find out things like where the bullet was or what its path was? I felt as if there was a time to proceed and a time to back off and let the team concentrate on

101

saving the person. We were supposed to be the AOC's eyes and ears on the unit, yet many times the AOC completely disregarded what we told them and directed us to do what they wanted us to do. So I called the medical examiner back, found out exactly what the concerns were and started to gather as much information as I could. Unfortunately that meant I had to wake the trauma surgeon. Once he was awake he decided to come down to the ICU and see what was going on. I apologized for waking him and he said in no uncertain terms that he would like to focus on saving the patient, not meeting the needs of the medical examiner. I told him I agreed but my AOC did not. I ended up moving my laptop into a back conference room so the team could concentrate on saving the patient. They would come and find me if they needed me.

In the morning I updated all the lab results for the TC who relieved me. They had given him 72 units of blood in less than 12 hours and hundreds of liters of IV fluid. He made it through the night though. And the next time I went to that hospital he was still there in the ICU but doing better, the last time I went they said he had been discharged into a rehab hospital. I have encountered at least two patients since I have been in my current job in home healthcare who, I'm sure, with their injuries and level of brain damage were evaluated as donors but taken off our radar when they didn't progress to brain death. Their family chose to do a tracheotomy and a feeding tube and they survived and are living, breathing, walking, talking, functioning people today.

■

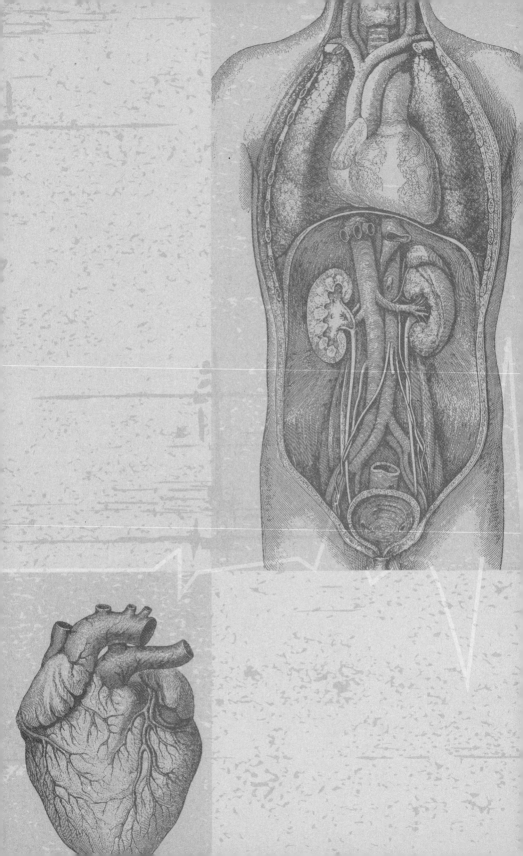

8

Will this Case Ever End?

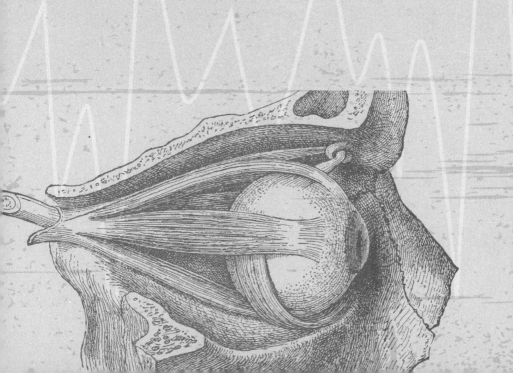

I T WAS FRIDAY; I WAS UP AT 5:30 A.M. CHECKING OUR PATIENT DATABASE TO see where I might be going that day. At 5:55 a.m. my initials, TLG, popped up next to a case at a hospital near the shore. I hopped in the shower, called my coworker who was already there and let her know when I would be there. Then I called my Administrator on Call to let them know I was on the way. With the traffic, I knew it would take me over two hours of driving to get there, so I settled in for the long drive, listening to music as usual. Once I arrived I grabbed my bags and walked into the hospital. Once I was on the trauma Intensive Care Unit my coworker gave me a report: the patient was a middle-aged mentally handicapped male, a ward of the state, no living relatives, lived in a group home and choked on his sandwich the previous night at dinner. No one there knew what to do and by the time help arrived he had been without oxygen long enough for his brain to be severely damaged. This is called a hypoxic injury during which the dead brain tissue makes fluid that presses down on the brain, causing brain death. Brain cells cannot regenerate after being deprived of oxygen. The patient was showing signs of progressing to full brain death and, once my coworker left to go home, I began to concentrate on getting him through that process without coding.

We were well trained to recognize the progression of brain death and we knew what signs and symptoms donors started to show when heading toward it. Reflexes seem to be lost in a certain order, the brain dies from the top down and the last part to go is the brain stem that controls all our really important life-sustaining functions like our heartbeat, our ability to maintain a blood pressure and our ability to breathe. It was not uncommon for us to be called when patients still had several reflexes. The worst-case scenario for us was that the patient survived and we shredded the paperwork, which of course was the best case scenario for the patient and always the outcome we hoped for.

I've seen some absolutely unbelievable efforts by trauma teams to save lives. When there is pressure inside the skull from either blood or fluid and it isn't relieved surgically, the patient's brain will eventually herniate, in other words be pushed down into the brain stem and cervical spine through the hole in the bottom of our skull called the foramen magnum. Once that happens the patient will no longer have any reflexes and will be unable to maintain their blood pressure. We were trained to get patients through this period; if a donor is going to become grossly unstable this is the time when it will happen. Usually overbreathing the ventilator was the last reflex to go as the area of the brain that controls breathing lies in the last part of the brain stem. Even ventilator-dependent patients retain the ability to take a few breaths on their own, even if it's only one or two every few minutes.

In this case, I huddled with the nurse; there was so much work to be done on the patient moving forward as a possible donor that we required a one-on-one assignment. This meant that the ICU nurse working with us would not have any other patients that had been promised by all our hospitals. I needed the nurse's help because Transplant Coordinators did not provide direct patient care, we did donor management like a critical care physician. We needed to get an IV placed immediately into a major vessel close to the heart for direct delivery of life-sustaining medications if we were going to get him through herniation without coding. These lines are placed by first accessing the vein with a large needle and feeding a guide wire through the vein down toward the heart. An IV catheter is slid over the guide wire, which is then removed, leaving the catheter in place. There is a pretty common complication, called a pneumothorax, that results from having lines like these placed. It occurs when the lung is pierced by the wire during placement and sometimes we would only find out that the lung had been pierced when the donor became difficult to ventilate. Central lines were often placed by residents so this problem was not uncommon. Thankfully the residents all knew how to fix it by placing a chest tube immediately into the cavity between the lung and chest wall that allowed the air that was displacing the deflated lung to escape and the lung to reinflate, eventually sealing off the leak. Every donor also required an arterial blood line, A-lines as they are called, usually placed in the radial artery in the wrist. They are a more effective and accurate way of measuring blood pressure than a blood pressure cuff that could be off by as much as 10 points. If your blood pressure is only 60/40, those are a very important 10 points. Not just anyone can place an A-line and in my experience the best are the anesthesiologists. Of course it's not always easy if you are somewhere that has no OR staff at night to call in the on-call anesthesiologist to do an arterial line on a donor. For this patient, I also requested they get some of the medications we used to support the blood pressure, called vasopressors, ready and hanging spiked at the bedside. I needed to make sure the crash cart was close by and accessible, this patient had a perfectly healthy liver and kidneys and we wanted to get them transplanted. Crash carts or code carts are universal in every hospital, they hold all drugs, IV's and breathing tubes needed in a cardiac or respiratory emergency, all in one place.

Thankfully, the central line that went directly into his vascular system was in place when he finally progressed. As predicted, his blood pressure dropped into the 50/30 level and we started with one vasopressor on a high drip rate, we would add them as needed during this period. Sometimes we had to use three or four vasopressors until we got things under control, then we could remove them one at a time. This was a critical time. We would do almost anything to get past this point and into brain death testing, including chest compressions if a family requested it, but not CPR because the intent was not to "resuscitate" the patient but to preserve the organs for donation. We were very aware that some of the terms we used could be confusing to the donor's family or misunderstood by the staff. We tried to keep the process as impersonal as possible and so we were not allowed to talk to the donor. I know that may sound nuts but most nurses do talk to their patients, even the unresponsive ones, but we never did that and would discourage the bedside nurse from doing it as well. Once the patient was pronounced, they were legally dead. During a class once, I did share with my boss that I had done autopsies for hospital pathologists for a couple years and I even talked to those patients — she was not amused.

The patient made it successfully through that process and had no reflexes left. I got the ball rolling to get pronouncement, the residents would decide whether to do a brain flow study or exams. Either way I had tons of work to do. The first challenge at the top of my list was finding a responsible party who would sign the consent form and answer the questions in the medical and social history we did for every donor. If you've ever donated blood it's very similar to that questionnaire. We could not allocate organs without getting this form completed. I started with calls to the home where the patient had lived and was lucky enough to get the medical director who went over the form with me. He wanted me to contact the state-appointed guardian to get consent, though. Great, get a state employee on a Friday afternoon, yeah right. I thanked the medical director for his help and promised to send him a letter with the outcome. I called the state agency that had been responsible for the patient and explained who I was and the reason for my call. The receptionist said she would contact the guardian and have her call me. While I waited I had a huge list of stuff to do, starting with updating lab results and faxing them over to my office. The blood type was required in duplicate from two different labs, the hospital lab and our independent lab that did the serology testing for infectious diseases. We had our own chart to maintain and we had to stay in constant communication with the AOC and with our office while they did the kidney allocation. The lists of people who needed kidneys were very long and the matching complicated. It took too much concentration to allocate them for the job to be done by someone who was constantly interrupted, like the TC onsite. When they completed the kidney allocation there was literally a "lineup" of potential recipients about 12 people long, who could be anywhere in the country since kidneys can survive out of the body for 48 hours.

The office required hourly updates on lab results that closely monitored the kidney function and what we nurses call "I and O's," or intake and output of fluids. It was crucial in good donor management to monitor the fluid intake verses the urine or stomach contents output so we didn't cause damage to the heart, lungs or kidneys. The heart and lung surgeons usually preferred the patient to be what they called "open and dry," meaning the lungs are open and not bogged down with excess fluids. You can tax the heart with too much fluid as well. On the other hand, the kidney surgeons liked lots of flushing to sort of clean out the kidneys and keep them functioning well. It was up to the TC to find a balance between these. I also had to get clearance from the medical examiner who told us if they were taking the case and if they had any restrictions or requests. The medical examiner decided if they would take any of our donors after the organ recovery for criminal investigation purposes. We called them for every patient and gave them the information we had found. If the medical examiner wanted to take an extra look after we were done we would get them tubes of blood before the recovery, obtain a tube of the patient's admission blood if possible and send them with the body. We had an excellent rapport with the medical examiners in our region and they would go to great lengths to assist us in making donation happen. Early on in this job I created a checklist for myself with every possible thing I would have to do from start to finish on a case. It's five pages long!

As I was doing all this they decided to take the patient down to nuclear medicine for a brain flow study. It was getting late in the day and I still hadn't heard from the guardian. In the state I was in, the law said that if the patient had no family the hospital administration could sign the consent form. This patient definitely couldn't lie there until Monday that was for sure. His liver function looked good from all the lab results, sometimes the liver enzymes rise after an episode with no oxygen, but as long as they were trending back down the liver was transplantable. Liver function can also affect the sodium levels and the ability for the donor to clot their own blood. Just like your ankles retain fluid with a salty diet, so does your liver. If a donor's sodium level is above 150 mEq/L, the normal range being 135-145 mEq/L, they can have what is called a "boggy liver," it's soft instead of firm and dense like it should be. We routinely gave patients a drug called mannitol at the time of incision in the OR. By the time the surgeons got to the liver the drug would have sucked all the excess fluid out caused by the sodium.

Finally, it was 4:30 p.m. when the guardian called the unit. I explained to her what had happened, who I was and what I needed from her. She was not happy, just did not want to be bothered. I told her how his kidneys and liver could save three lives that night and his corneas could give a blind person sight, but I couldn't do it without her. So she agreed and I told her I would call her right back. The office could record a three-way telephone call and in this way we could have a witness to the consent. We called her back and I went through the consent process. If a patient does not have donor designation on their license or state identification then we needed to ask for each organ individually. The consenting individual is required to say yes or no to each one. The list we requested was: heart, lungs, liver, kidneys, pancreas, intestines, bone, skin, tendons, vertebral bodies, ribs, heart for valves if not being transplanted, corneas and whole eyes. Imagine asking someone for each of those things one after another. It's one of the hardest things I've ever done.

As soon as I was done obtaining consent I updated my AOC. The patient was due back from nuclear medicine any time now, the preliminary read (the unofficial results) had been called up to me as "no flow," meaning the patient had no blood flow to his brain. The medical examiner had given clearance for liver, kidneys and tissue. I ran down my list of "to-do" stuff and told him I would talk to him when I had an OR time. I started allocating the liver, a healthy liver surely someone would want it. The donor did test positive for Hepatitis B but it was not active. I started my liver calls and the very first surgeon on the list from a nearby inner-city hospital interrupted my explanation and said, "I'll take it, if I don't my patient will die. Call me with an OR time." Great, I called the OR and asked for an approximate time and told them we were going to take just the liver, kidneys and tissue afterward. This hospital was a level 1 Trauma Center and they were busy at all times of the night. The charge nurse said she felt I could arrange for a 7 a.m. start time. I looked at the clock and cringed knowing I would not being getting any relief and would have to stay until the OR was done. "OK, if I can go any earlier let me know." I said. As I was making these calls I watched as a few of the patients' caretakers from the group home came in to say their goodbyes. They said he was a sweet man and was loved by all at the home. I promised to send them an outcome letter in about two weeks.

I spoke with the perfusionist from our office to confirm her arrival time; sometimes we had them pick up some of the recipient surgeons in hospitals close to the office. They are all usually fellows who intend to be transplant surgeons and are on their donor rotation or senior residents on a transplant rotation. Whenever kidneys and liver are both being recovered the liver transplant program will also take out the kidneys. Our perfusionist would pack them in ice and either take them to the office to be pumped for 24 to 48 hours or to one of the local transplant centers. Sometimes we had couriers come for them as well. On this particular night my recovery surgeon was visiting his mother and he drove down in about two hours.

Things seemed to be going smoothly, the OR time was set for 7:00 a.m., according to the nursing supervisor they had a fractured wrist to repair scheduled for 7 a.m. as well, but were going to bump him back on the schedule. She didn't feel it was necessary to call and wake the orthopedic surgeon in the middle of the night to tell him his wrist fracture was being moved back. She said she would call him between 5:00 a.m. and 5:30 a.m. and I continued on with all the last-minute stuff that remained to be done. I had to ensure we had complete copies of the chart to go with each recipient organ and had to double- and triple-check to make sure I had all required signatures. Then I had to update and fax my last morning lab results to the office, call and update my AOC and run through the recipient lineup. The liver was allocated locally but backed up locally, regionally and nationally, which was our policy. A liver can get declined intraoperatively for quality, a biopsy result or size, so to make sure it didn't go to waste we would have several surgeons waiting in the wings, telling them I would call if they became primary. The last few backups would be from what we called aggressive liver programs, they have the sickest patients and will frequently take a substandard liver and do a bridge transplant. They will use it until they can find a better one, but at least the patient doesn't die and we don't waste a liver. There was lots of communication between myself and the liver recipient surgeon because the recipient needed to have dialysis just before heading to the OR. He was in kidney failure as well, but they hoped his kidneys would start working again with his new liver. This was a common scenario with liver failure patients. If the kidneys didn't start working again, the patient would be placed on the kidney list. Although it doesn't seem to make much sense at times, the industry is seriously and strictly regulated. By that point my perfusionist was on her way, my surgeon was on his way, the recipient was heading to dialysis and the donor was stable.

I took a few minutes to gather my thoughts and went to change into scrubs thinking how this man had no living family but after the donation, he would have a family. A family who may not know his name, may not know how sweet and childlike he was, but who would never forget him and would always credit him with saving their life. I went and had a fresh cup of coffee; the nurses would frequently make sure we always had hot, fresh coffee — thankfully! Sometimes during quiet moments like that I would try and imagine how the recipient must have felt. How do you handle knowing someone died but that you can live? How do you handle knowing a body part from someone who has died is being placed into your body?

Around 5:45 a.m. I made a call down to the OR charge nurse just to make sure we were still running on time. The surgical tech (which is the job I did for 16 years before becoming a nurse) informed me that the orthopedic surgeon had found out he was "being bumped for an organ harvest" and he moved his case up to 6:45 a.m.; saying that I went nuts was probably an understatement. Things really started to go downhill from there, the nursing supervisor showed up to tell me the surgeon was mad that she bumped him without calling and he was on his way into the hospital. I tried several frantic times to call my AOC but he wouldn't answer, there was one AOC that was well known for disappearing and I had to be on call with him for that case! I asked the ICU nurse and respiratory therapist if they were ready to go, they packed up all his lines and monitor and said they were. My Blackberry rang and it was the recovery surgeon, who usually arrived in scrubs with other residents or with perfusion. This time he had shown up alone in jeans and a t-shirt; he was calling to tell me he was there and I heard the OR nurse arguing with him in the background. I yelled at him, "Tell her you're the surgeon for Christ's sake!" I picked up the unit phone, called the OR and said, "We are on our way down." They tried to tell me they were starting the wrist and I would have to wait for the second team to get in. I said, "I didn't ask you if I could come down, I said I'm coming down. Now." I had put in too many hours and the recipient timing was crucial, I wasn't going to be pushed back for a wrist fracture that had been in the hospital for three days already just because the orthopedic surgeon wanted the rest of his Saturday to be free.

I tried my AOC at least three times on the way to the OR, no answer. We walked through the OR doors (the surgeon later jokingly said I "stormed through" the door, I won't deny I was pissed, not to mention completely exhausted) and were greeted by anesthesia, the nurse anesthetist looked confused and everyone was arguing. I insisted we be put in an OR room so the donor could be properly monitored and ventilated. Finally they agreed and took him into a room down the hall from all the ruckus. I was trying to focus on all the things I had to do now that we'd entered the OR, unlike the majority of my fellow TC's I was very comfortable in the OR because of my background. It was a little like being on a different planet where they spoke a foreign language. There were things to review with anesthesia: drugs, and when to give them, dosages, a reminder to not give the lethal dose of heparin until I told him to (not when the surgeon said to give it, only when I said to give it). We gave 300 units per kilogram about five minutes before cross clamping the aorta and vena cava, it thinned the blood so the liver and kidneys didn't get congested with blood clots. You would never give that much heparin to a living patient, not unless you wanted to kill them. The circulating nurse came in and said, "Who's the transplant coordinator?" Someone pointed at me and she said, "Doctor wants to see you in the hall."

Oh god. One thing I knew about surgeons was they liked to kick the dead horse so to speak. I used to work with an OR nurse who would say to them sometimes, "See that dead horse in the corner? Quit kicking it!" They just couldn't let go of things and the surgeon was loaded and ready to attack. I walked out in the hall, he was a 6' 4" Indian man with a full, dark beard, quite intimidating, but I wasn't in any mood to play games. "What's up?" I said as I walked into the lounge where he was waiting. He started telling me how furious he was that I had just come down here with no notice and now he would have to wait. I explained to him that I had been there since yesterday working on this donor and the nursing supervisors had known I would be going to the OR in the morning since late the previous night. They chose not to call and wake him but instead waited until about 5 a.m. to call and tell him he was not starting at 7 a.m. as scheduled, none of which I had any control over. I told him that I wasn't so happy, nor would hospital administration be too happy when they found out how he tried to sneak his way into the OR before me without any regard for timing on our side. He didn't care, as he yelled at me a male nurse was writing my name down on a piece of paper from my ID badge. When he told me that he did a rotation in transplant and I was not even guaranteed these organs would be transplanted I said to him, "this conversation is over" and walked away. Back to the room for more chaos. The recipient surgeon sent a very new medical student to help the surgeon and, as I walked in the room, he was in the process of getting his ass chewed out by yet another OR nurse. I said under my surgical mask, "what the hell is wrong with this place?" Again I tried my AOC, getting nothing. This was unbelievable, they could be up your ass all case and when I needed him the most he wasn't answering for over an hour. I was so exhausted I felt like crying, which happens sometimes when you have worked for more than 24 hours straight with no sleep, and we hadn't even made an incision yet! The surgeon prepped and draped, I gave pathology a call to make sure he had arrived for the liver and kidney biopsies we would need. I called my AOC, finally he answered, I stretched the phone cord out into the sub sterile area and told him what had been happening. His only words were, "Hold your ground." At least I knew I wasn't in trouble. As I sat down in the OR room to get caught up on my own paperwork someone walked in the room and said, "Who's the transplant coordinator"? I dropped my head into my hands and mumbled, "I am." She identified herself as the chief of anesthesia — oh great, she came in on a Saturday morning just to yell at me. She surprised me by saying she wanted to reaffirm the hospital's commitment to making donation a reality whenever they could, which made me finally start to relax. Other than the orthopedic surgeon acting like a clown there were no more problems, the rest of the case went smoothly. The liver and kidneys looked great and were on their way to their new homes.

I walked out of the hospital around 2 p.m. in search of a hotel room. I had arrived around 8 a.m. the day before. As always I parked on the roof; a hotel is attached to the hospital here so I literally drove to the other side and staggered into the hotel lobby, dragging my bag with my company credit card in hand. Not much longer I kept telling myself. I got up to the desk, I told the girl I needed a room, any room, for most of the day. She said, "We're booked. In fact the whole city is booked, there's a Corvette convention." I was stunned speechless for about 30 seconds and then started to lose it, sobbing the whole way back to the car, not caring who was watching me. I had a total meltdown in the car. It's like all the emotion you control overnight comes out, all at once, all the sadness and frustration just spill out all over the place with no filters. I called my husband and state that I am driving home. He said that's probably not smart but knows better than to argue with me when I'm like this. I did try and make it home, but my brain took over and when it saw one of those hotel signs on the side of the highway I pulled off. It was a total dump but all I needed was a bed, a bathroom and air conditioning. I slept for about five hours, got up, showered and made coffee. I drove home, wondering what the outcome would be for this recipient. He was not Hepatitis B positive but was accepting the liver anyway so he could live. They were going to treat him with medications for the Hepatitis he would get from the donor. About a week later, I was on call and heading into one of our frequented city hospital transplant centers. It suddenly dawned on me that the liver recipient would be up on this unit so I asked the chief resident. He pointed into a room across from the nurse's desk and there sat a man across from his wife, eating lunch together, laughing and talking. The resident said, "There's the person you worked all those hours for the other night. He's about to be transferred to the step-down unit." Seeing him there with his wife made it all worthwhile. He was someone's husband, father, brother, uncle or grandfather and they would have him a little longer because of something I did.

■

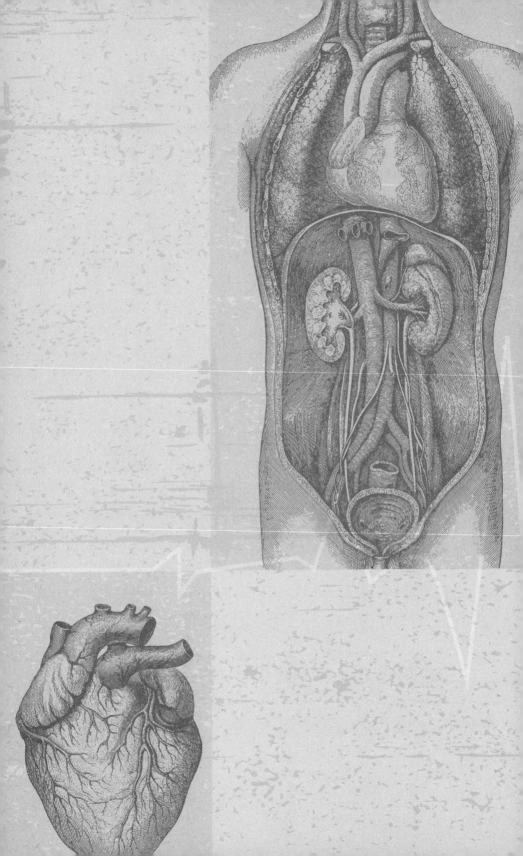

9

Dual
Advocacy

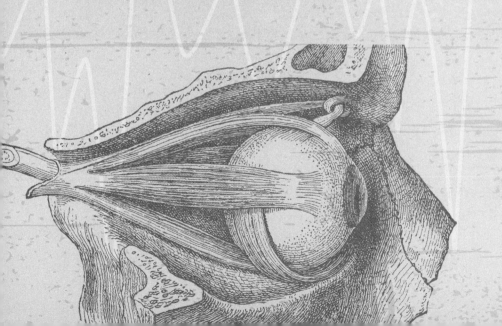

ANOTHER CASE I WAS INVOLVED IN WAS VERY CHALLENGING AND COULD easily be perceived by some as unethical. This is how this case unfolded and how the neurosurgeon gave a grieving family a very rare opportunity to make educated decisions about the patient's end of life by just being honest with them. It was the start of 48 hours on call and I was headed out to a large hospital on the city limits. The patient was a 68-year-old Korean female who had suffered a large hemorrhagic stroke a few days earlier. In other words, she was bleeding in her brain but she was not brain dead yet. She had two sons and a husband with her at the hospital, holding a constant bedside vigil. This always made it difficult for the Transplant Coordinators because we needed to get in the room and examine the patient but we couldn't do that if the family was in the room. Many times we would wait until the nurses went in to do something like clean the patient up, they would ask the family to step out and we would sneak into the room. As I have said before, we walked a very fine line sometimes between being ethical and unethical in our practice.

This lady had come in a few days earlier and the family had decided to let the neurosurgeon perform a procedure called a craniotomy. This involves drilling a hole through the skull to relieve the pressure building up against the brain from the bleeding. In some brain-injured patients that are expected to have significant brain swelling, the neurosurgeons will take off a "flap" of bone from the skull, leaving a small window into the brain.

The piece of bone that is removed is wrapped in sterile, moist gauze and placed into a sterile jar, labeled and usually kept in the fridge that holds medications in the Operating Room (OR). Many times the neurosurgeons place a drain called a Lycox that measures pressure inside the skull. The Lycox is hooked up to a monitor that continuously gives a pressure reading. People with high intracranial pressures will progress to brain death very quickly without intervention. People with massive brain injuries who have intervention sometimes will get into that terrible scenario of having no chance of a meaningful recovery but will not progress to brain death. In the case of this woman, considering her age, her only chance to be a donor was brain death and her intracranial pressures had been stable since she came out of the OR. Her only reflexes were overbreathing the ventilator, which meant she was very close to death. Ventilators are set with a respiratory rate and volume based on a calculation using a patient's height and weight. If the ventilator is set to breathe 16 times a minute and you look on the monitor to see the patient is breathing 22 times a minute, they are overbreathing the ventilator. Breathing is usually the last reflex a patient loses.

In most of the hospitals we frequented neurosurgeons were not always thrilled to see us and sometimes made our jobs very difficult. We only came when they couldn't save the patient. Unfortunately we needed them because most brain death policies stated at least one examination must be done by a neurologist or neurosurgeon, so we had to deal with them. Thankfully, at this particular hospital we had an excellent relationship with the chief of neurosurgery. He had even spoken at many of our educational seminars for healthcare providers. I was very happy to see he was my attending physician although I had no idea what he was about to do.

As was our normal practice I contacted him as soon as I had arrived to let him know I was there. You never wanted to surprise a neurosurgeon with your presence on the Intensive Care Unit (ICU) by evaluating his patient, although it happened to all of us at one time or another. You get there and get tied up in either donor instability or some family issues and don't get to them before they see you, which is never good. He answered the page and told me he would be right up, "don't move" he said. I busied myself gathering lab results from the computer system at the hospital, yet another thing that was difficult at some hospitals. Nurses are strictly warned to never let another person log in under their name and I would frequently have to go into my dissertation that I would never risk my own license by documenting under their name. Most agreed that sounded reasonable. Some places actually gave us our own log-ins and passwords. There was always something to do when starting a case, lab results needed to be recorded from admission up until that point and faxed to the office, blood plasma volumes needed to be calculated, intake and output were added up and you would need to assess what is going on with the family. Once the chief of neurosurgery arrived he sat down next to me at the desk and started telling me what he knew about the patient and the family. He knew that culturally this husband, who only spoke Korean, would have a very difficult time making the decision to withdraw support from his wife. He knew that she had zero chance of recovery and if they chose to trach and peg her she would end up dying a miserable death in some state-funded nursing home.

This is a decision many families have to make, if a patient is on a ventilator for too long the endotracheal tube, or breathing tube, will literally erode through the trachea. If a patient's life is going to be sustained the family will need to consent to a feeding tube being placed, which is commonly referred to as a "peg tube or g tube." It's essentially a tube placed directly into the patient's stomach through the abdominal wall that nutrients and medications are fed through. You can't stay on IV's forever. The chief brought me up to speed, telling me he personally had checked all her other reflexes and they were gone; she only had taken a couple breaths over the ventilator every few minutes, which is enough to prevent brain death pronouncement. Her Lycox pressures had been stable and it was still actively draining, which would become an important part of the scenario about to unfold. He suggested we meet with the family together, just he and I, the patient's sons would translate for their father. We were strongly discouraged from using a family member to translate because we were never really sure what was being said, so I contacted the hospital interpreters and they had a Korean man come up to the unit. I spoke with him briefly, explaining as best I could what the conversation would be about while the doctor gathered the family in a conference room. It was always refreshing and inspiring to see a physician who was able to humbly admit that, despite his best efforts, he had been unable to save the patient but felt there at least there was something he could give the family—the gift of donation.

We all went into the room and I made sure we had water and tissues, multiple boxes, they were a staple when having family conversations and we had been trained to have everything we would need so the family could have our undivided attention. I remember thinking it was dumb asking if they needed anything when we did role-playing in training. Then, suddenly, you were with a real family—one that had suffered some kind of tragedy—and the situation would be so emotionally difficult that you would never remember those little things if you weren't trained to do them. Everyone sat down, the room was set up for a medical teaching conference with tables arranged in a large rectangle with chairs on the outside. The physician took a chair and broke through the tables to sit directly across from the husband. The sons sat on either side of their father, next to one son was the nurse and next to the other was the translator. I sat at the first chair along the side next to the translator so we were in a kind of "L" shape with the doctor in the center. He opened the conversation by saying how sorry he was that we had to have such a talk on that day and that he had tried everything he knew to save the patient, but that goal had become impossible. Every time he spoke it was followed by the hospital interpreter translating into Korean.

The husband looked absolutely exhausted, as if his life was slipping away along with hers, it was very sad. The doctor presented them with three options. Option one was to make her comfortable and withdraw support. According to the sons, just as predicted, culturally this was not an option as it was not considered a natural death. Option two was to trach, peg and move the woman into long-term care, this was not something the physician recommended. Option three was to clamp off her Lycox drain, allow her intracranial pressures to rise enough for her to progress to brain death, which would allow her to be an organ donor. I thought to myself, "Wait, what did he just say? Did I hear him correctly?" He went on to explain to the family that brain death is a natural death that is inevitable and irreversible. He also explained to them that the single thing that prevented her progression to brain death was that Lycox drain. The family was silent, taking in every word he said. He then told a personal story about a young girl he knew who had died waiting for a heart transplant, and how he felt watching the girl's father cry openly at her funeral while he spoke of never walking his daughter down the aisle, never holding her children, never seeing her again except in his memories. Everyone in the room was crying now, including the attending physician. I still consider this the best example of what we called dual advocacy; helping the family make the right decision that was best for them, while still being an advocate for the recipients. It took a lot of guts and confidence for this doctor to pull it off, yet he did it flawlessly. They agreed, Option three was for them. They shared with us how their mom was so giving and generous, constantly tending to their every need while they were growing up. She had given selflessly in life to her family, her church and her Korean community and now she would continue that giving into her death. This was a closure they could all live with and accept.

I finished the necessary paperwork with the family, updated my office and Administrator on Call (AOC), and went to find the attending to discuss what would happen overnight. He would clamp off her Lycox sometime later that night, he ordered an arterial IV line be placed for close monitoring of blood pressure and placed all the necessary orders for the medications the nurses would need to support her blood pressure through herniation. He expected they would start the first exam in the morning. I was sent home and informed I would go back the next day to finish the case. I placed our own chart in the slot with the hospital chart and headed home. As I was driving my pager went off. Oh God, now what? I called the office and they said the patient's son had called and would like to speak with me.

I hung up and called his cell phone. He told me they had failed to discuss an important detail about their culture and now his father was considering rescinding consent. He explained that if his mother could not be buried whole or complete as a donor, they would not want to donate. If she was to be buried "intact," they had no problem with donation. I was stunned. I pulled over, asked him if I could call him back in a few minutes, that I wanted to confirm something. I called my AOC and told him the scenario, he quickly explained to me that most, if not all, of the major organs are removed in order to embalm someone, and in the U.S. if you are being transported across state lines or if you are being buried you had to be embalmed. I told him I thought that was true but wanted to confirm it with him before telling the son, "but how will I tell him that?" I asked. My AOC said, "You have more than enough training to handle this situation, you can do this." I called the son back and as gently and vaguely as I could tried to explain the embalming process to him. He continued to ask a lot of questions, like how do they get the organs out if they make no large incisions? Somehow I managed to explain that the organs were removed in pieces, silently praying he didn't ask how they did that, he didn't ask, thank god. I really did not want to explain to him that the funeral director will insert large tubings or cannulas into a couple major blood vessels and he will flush out the blood and replace it with embalming fluids. The organs are cut into smaller pieces with a large hook and then flushed out, sometimes they add embalming fluid or filler to the abdominal cavity once they are removed so the skin doesn't sink in and decomposition doesn't occur. The son was satisfied that he could calm his father's fears with that answer and agreed we would meet at the hospital in the morning.

The next day I was up at 5 a.m. and out the door by 6 a.m., knowing I had a long day and night ahead of me. I got to the hospital, gathered my things and headed into the unit. I walked into the patient's room and sure enough, her intracranial pressures had been climbing since the Lycox was clamped and she was having trouble supporting her blood pressure. The nurses already had her on two vasopressors going through the central line to help support her blood pressure. She had herniated not long before I arrived, had stopped overbreathing the ventilator and the nurses had already alerted the physician, who was on his way in. The family arrived with coffee and donuts for the staff and they gave a couple of beautiful floral arrangements from her room to the nurses to take home. Once the neurosurgeon arrived he confirmed she had stopped overbreathing the ventilator and got ready to perform the first brain death exam with the family in the room. This was always a powerful time and for most families was the defining moment in their acknowledgment that their loved one was gone from this world. Not all doctors were comfortable doing this in front of the family but for the ones that were, it was an incredible step toward acceptance of the death for the grieving family. I stood quietly in the back of the room while the doctor performed the universal exams for brain death as the patient's husband sat next to her, holding her hand. He even explained to them how her eyes would roll around as he moved her head, explaining while he did it which cranial nerves were making that happen. Looking at her arterial blood gas results we would need to do some work to get her normalized in her acid-base balance in order to do an apnea test. In the meantime they were scheduling her to go to nuclear medicine for a cerebral blood flow study. I huddled with the nurse and respiratory therapist about how we could maximize her lungs and normalize her blood gas results so we could do the apnea test after the blood flow study. Both nurses had some great ideas and we agreed to start changing some of her ventilator settings.

Arterial blood gases are complicated to explain, but basically the body has two systems responsible for maintaining our acid-base balance, which is essential for life, the metabolic system (the kidneys) and the respiratory system (the lungs). A patient can be in either respiratory acidosis or alkalosis or metabolic acidosis or alkalosis. The lab results of arterial blood samples tell you which is happening. There are four components to an arterial blood gas and depending on which is up or down you can tell if the patient's condition is metabolic or respiratory in origin, which in turn tells you how to correct the problem. Most of the time if a patient is in metabolic acidosis it can be corrected by giving sodium bicarbonate. If a patient is in respiratory alkalosis you can adjust the ventilator setting, allowing the patient to either retain or exhale more CO_2. Think of it as a chemistry equation with elements that need to be in balance, if the body can't achieve balance alone we have to help it along. This process can take hours and hours of changes before you get it right, you could only change one thing at a time, then redraw the arterial blood gas and reassess the results and, as usual, you would have about one thousand other things to do. When this patient came back from the blood flow study we were able to do the apnea. She was pronounced and the family was informed of her time of death. They said their goodbyes to the staff, ensured I had correct contact information and left with the husband looking as if a 100-pound weight had been lifted from his shoulders. I promised to call later and send them a letter with the outcome of the donations in about two weeks.

The physician helped enter all my necessary orders into the computer system for the testing we needed to evaluate her organs. We ordered an echocardiogram, usually called an "echo" (an ultrasound of the heart and valves), a bronchoscopy (where the doctor uses a flexible scope to look at the lungs from the inside) and a cardiac catheterization if the echo result was good. To complicate matters both the echo team and the pulmonologist to do the bronchoscopy showed up at exactly the same time, which did not go over very well. The pulmonary doctor was pissed, but I have a knack for diffusing doctors and it worked on him like a charm. He asked why I had ordered the test so early. I explained that I was trying to avoid something they all hated: making him come back to the hospital late at night to evaluate a donor for us. That seemed to satisfy him. He left and said he would be back in an hour. It was our normal practice to start out evaluating every organ. The echocardiogram produces a result that is called the "ejection fraction," this is a percentage calculation based on numerous measurements within the heart that equate to the heart's ability to effectively pump blood to the rest of the body. An ejection fraction of 65 percent or better is required to transplant the heart and if the result is at least 65 percent you can proceed with a cardiac catheterization to look for arterial blockages in the heart. This patient's heart did not meet the criteria for transplant so we cancelled the cardiac catheterization and moved forward with the bronchoscopy of the lungs.

I had been communicating with a lung transplant coordinator at an inner-city program who had a recipient that was interested. Most of the centers I contacted had declined due to the donor's age but this program had an older recipient who was a match. She requested I draw arterial blood gases every two hours with every other set being after what we called an O_2 challenge. Our practice was to draw them every four hours, correct as needed and do O_2 challenges if we were not getting good results. An O_2 challenge involves turning up the pressure on the ventilator that keeps the lungs open at a cellular level, it can maximize lung function and make the difference between lungs being transplanted or wasted. It's literally like an exercise for the lungs. This is a busy time and you have to watch closely how much fluid the patient is getting because the lungs can't be wet, they have to be "open and dry" and that means monitoring kidney function closely. Sometimes the donor needs blood products to either help with clotting issues or to replace the volume of blood being lost from drawing off hundreds of tubes for testing and matching. In that case, I thought it would be better to be flexible and do what the recipient surgeon wanted, which meant doing arterial blood gases every two hours instead of every four and getting the lungs placed. My AOC did not, it turned out, agree with my thought process.

The lung coordinator had told me the recipient would be flying down from another state up north and had a chartered plane basically on standby all the time waiting for this moment. The recipient went into the OR at the same time as the donor, so timing was crucial. Some of the results coming back were not as good as I had hoped and the bronchoscopy showed her lungs were red and excoriated inside. I reported these results to my AOC and he started questioning me about doing arterial blood gases every two hours. He got very angry and started yelling at me that I needed to "remember what team I play for and who signs my paycheck." He said I should not take orders from a lung coordinator and I should not be giving them the bad results. I was shocked. "You want me to only report the good results?" He said, "Yes, if we can keep them interested long enough to come out and look at the lungs, they are more likely to take them." I could not believe what he was saying; these were human lungs, not a used car. There was a recipient getting on a plane to fly here thinking he was getting the lungs he had been waiting for and it was not fair to mislead him on the condition of the lungs. The nurses on the ICU could hear the AOC yelling at me on the desk phone and could see that I had started crying. I want to explain something, this particular AOC was very smart, even funny at times, but he was a jerk, a bully. He liked to play god and had let the high administrative position he held inflate his opinion of himself and it was ugly. I'm sure there may be others like him across the country but they are the minority. Most of the AOC's I worked with were truly dedicated individuals who were leaders in their field, locally and nationally. When on call they would be dealing with each one of the cases we were out on, anything going on at the office and any "fly outs," which are when our perfusionist went with a transplant team to recover an organ somewhere else. They were intimately involved in every aspect of a transplant. I had seen a few of them do extraordinary things on call when they came out on difficult cases to help. But this particular night it was all about following the AOC's orders and not the lung coordinator's. I had no choice, I did call the lung coordinator and let her know I could not do arterial blood gases every two hours, only every four hours, and she figured out on her own what was going on. She said it was no problem and the surgeon was going to come take a look so call when I set the OR time.

At 4 a.m. we ended up in the OR. The lung surgeon came since he was not far away, took one look with a scope and declined. I was extremely upset and he spent a considerable amount of time calming me down. He told me he understood who was behind the games that night and not to worry, he would explain to the recipient. Patients waiting for a transplant all knew that there was no guarantee they would wake up with a new pair of lungs and most had multiple false alarms. I still felt terrible about the whole thing. The donor did end up saving four lives that night. Her liver, two kidneys and her pancreas all changed lives. For me it was an incredible experience.

■

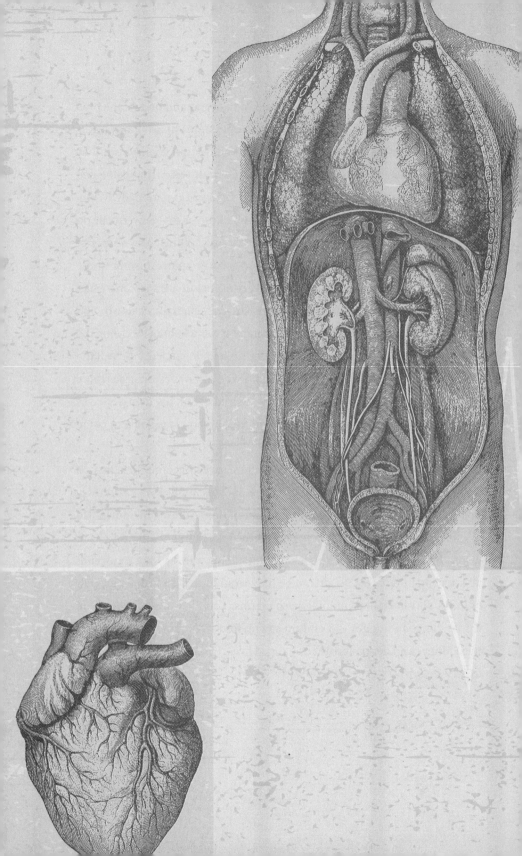

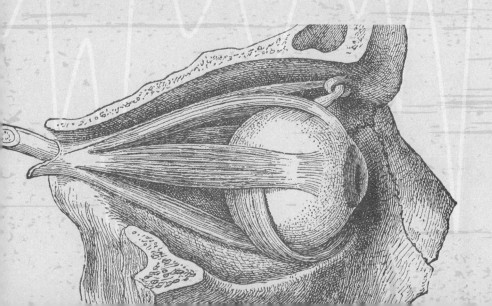

10

Example of
a Letter to a
Donor Family

THIS IS AN EXAMPLE OF A LETTER WE WOULD SEND TO THE DONOR FAMILY about two weeks after consent. We would go into the recipient database and look up the information that the recipient transplant centers had updated so we could tell the family as much as possible. A version of this letter would also sent to the president and CEO of the hospital where the donor died, the Intensive Care Unit involved, the Operating Room staff, sometimes to the hospital pathologists if they were involved doing biopsies and the medical examiner who gave clearance for donation.

Dear Mr. Smith:

I want to extend my deepest condolences to you for the loss of your mother. The sudden death of a loved one is one of the most painful experiences a family can endure. Your strength and courage in thinking of others during this difficult time are a tribute to you and to your mother's memory. I would like to share with you some information about the outcome of your mother's gifts.

The precious gift of your mother's liver was given to a 48-year-old single father of one daughter from the metropolitan area. Before he became ill he worked as a mechanic. He is still in the hospital due to an infection but is recovering nicely from the transplant. His liver function is good and he is looking forward to going home soon. He is so grateful for the transplant.

The gift of your mother's right kidney was given to a 60-year-old mother of three children also living in the metropolitan region. Before she got sick she worked in quality assurance in the mental health field. Her kidney failure was due to chronic high blood pressure and diabetes. She was discharged to go home on July 21st and is feeling great. She no longer requires dialysis and is looking forward to getting back to her busy lifestyle.

The gift of your mother's left kidney was given to a 57-year-old man with several children who lives in the area. His kidney failure was also due to chronic high blood pressure and diabetes. He was discharged to go home on July 22nd and no longer requires dialysis. He says he feels like he has a second chance at life because of the gift he received from your mom. He has been on disability since becoming ill but worked in the local post office before his kidneys failed. This patient reported to me that he is "making good urine," something we all take for granted but for him is the best indicator that he is doing well!

Your mother's corneas were recovered and gave the precious gift of sight to two women, a 66-year-old female from a neighboring state and a 59-year-old female from the area. These women entered the operating room blind and came out of surgery with the ability to see. They are extremely grateful.

Unfortunately, during our medical evaluation we found that your mother's heart, lungs, pancreas, intestines and tissues were not suitable for transplantation and therefore were not surgically recovered. Transplantation is about the hope that you give to people on the waiting list when you consent to donation. Thank you again for your commitment.

I want to remind you that you are not responsible for any hospital costs relating directly to organ donation. Unfortunately, on rare occasions, hospital billing errors do occur. If you receive a hospital bill that mistakenly includes charges relating to donation, please contact our finance department and they will help to correct the situation as soon as possible.

Although you are under no obligation to do so, you may write to the transplant recipients if you wish. I am enclosing a brochure entitled Writing to Transplant Recipients and Their Families that will guide you through the process.

I am also enclosing a booklet entitled For Those Who Give and Grieve and a brochure that describes the family support services available to you. One of our bereavement counselors will be contacting you shortly.

It was an honor to be able to fulfill your mother's last wish to be an organ donor and three lives were saved and two people have sight as a result. Although we met under very difficult circumstances, it was our pleasure to work with a family as close and caring as yours. On behalf of the Regional Organ Donor Program and the transplant recipients, please accept our sincerest gratitude for your generous gift. If you have any questions, please do not hesitate to call us at 1-800-XXX-XXXX.

Kindest Regards,

Traci Graf, RN, CST
Transplant Coordinator

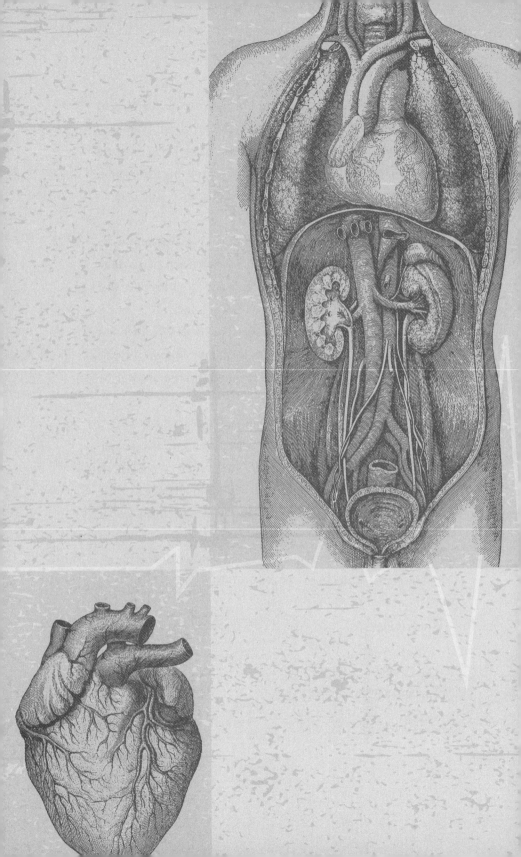

11

Pediatric Recovery

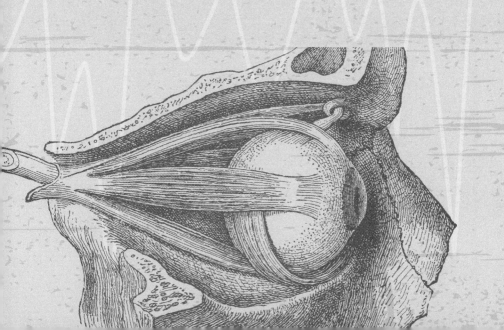

A T 6 A.M. MY PAGER WENT OFF. IT WAS MY FIRST DAY ON CALL AS PART OF A required 48-hour shift. I hated pediatrics and had been watching a case unfold on our constantly updated patient database since the night before, knowing there was a high potential I would be going there. I was already up and showered when I saw my initials, TLG, pop up next to my coworker's name, she had been there all night. I called the clinical phone coordinator back. We all took turns in this role, covering the phones, getting nonstop referrals for people near death and sending Transplant Coordinators all over the region at any time of night. As one of my bosses always said, "Transplant stops for nothing." Only one or two percent of all people who die can be organ donors and the number of actual donors is even smaller, so if the potential for organ donation was there, we went to check things out.

The clinical phone coordinator gave me my assignment for the day and I called my coworker onsite, got a quick report, told her how long it would take me to get there and hit the road. I usually listened to loud music to de-stress or talked to a fellow TC on her way somewhere else. There was considerable camaraderie among those of us on call together every day. Who else could you talk to at 3:30 a.m. when even your eighth cup of coffee wasn't working to keep you awake except someone in the same boat at another hospital. We were all chronic Blackberry messengers and stayed in close contact with each other at all hours of the night.

That morning was different though. I was headed to one of the largest and best-known pediatric hospitals in the world to take a three-month-old "shaken baby syndrome" donor to the Operating Room (OR) and I could think of nothing else. I kept thinking my coworker had already gotten consent so all I had to do was get the baby to the OR and we would be done. Infant donors are very rare and this baby's 18-year-old mother had graciously donated all the baby's organs. There were potentially five recipients whose lives were about to be changed forever as I made that drive.

I parked my car on the roof of the garage, a habit I started after being too tired to find my car one night in a garage, resulting in a total emotional meltdown. The hospital staff knew when we were there if they walked past our telltale "DONATE LIFE" license plates on a Honda civic. I got out and began to gather the supplies I would need from my trunk and packed them into my large rolling bag. I didn't think I would need too much since most of the work that required supplies happened during donor management when the organs were being allocated. I would need the culture tubes for the OR, my scrubs and my shoes. I continued to run through all the important details I would need to focus on to make this a successful recovery. I walked into the hospital, which can be a very long walk in the big inner-city hospital complexes. I went up to the Intensive Care Unit (ICU) and found two of my coworkers faxing last-minute labs to the office, making final copies of the chart for each recipient surgeon and directing the Registered Nurses (RN's) and anesthesia personnel who had come to transport the baby to the OR. We packed up and walked down the hall with the entire team all huddled around this tiny little ball of warm blankets with many tubes coming out of it. I saw no sign of the mother as she had said her goodbyes in the room, or that was what I assumed at that time. When we arrived in the OR there were a lot of people who swarmed around the baby, anesthesia staff mostly, everyone trying their hardest to keep her little body oxygenated and perfused for her organs. One of my coworkers started giving me the report while the other got acquainted with the OR staff and surgeons. The heart was going to the Maryland area and the lungs were going to New York State. Both of them were within a certain mile radius limit for how far they could be transported because they could only withstand being out of the body for four hours. The liver, pancreas and intestines were going to a large hospital in North Carolina, one recipient getting all three.

Each team required certain information, the surgeons needed to see the infectious disease testing results, the declaration of death including medical examiner clearance or restrictions, the blood typing by the hospital and the medical and social history done on every donor no matter the age. The surgeons had to sign a document before scrubbing to confirm they reviewed those four pieces of the chart. This could be a very busy, kind of crazy time. Lots of people, including fellows, residents and OR staff, needed to make sure they had the necessary transportation out of there, whether that be helicopters, planes or ambulances. These all needed to be on standby at an easily accessible exit. Once they cross clamped the aorta, every second counted.

My coworker finished her report, I was taking notes and trying to pay attention to what was happening with the donor too. My coworker then told me that she promised the mother and family that I would allow them to see the baby after the organ recovery. I stopped writing, looked at her, and said, "You're kidding me?" She said it would be fine; the hospital social worker would help me and then, completely exhausted, she and the other TC left.

We had a moment of silence for that little, lost life out of respect for the donor, something we all practiced and sometimes even had a picture to share from the family. The surgeons made the incision and things were under way. The heart team always went first, and then the lung, then the liver and/or pancreas, the kidneys came out last. The nurse anesthetist started reading from the chart what had happened to this little one, her 17-year-old father had shaken her in an effort to make her stop crying and instead caused irreversible damage to her little brain. The OR tended to be an area where some pretty heavy discussions occurred. I worked in an OR for 16 years handing instruments to surgeons so I was used to it, but that day was tough. The nurse anesthetist started to lose it, crying openly, apologizing to us for her inability to control her emotions. There were some strong opinions about what should happen to her father. I gave them a different perspective by pointing out the age of the parents and the fact that the 17-year-old dad probably had never even handled a baby her age before. He was turning himself into the police at the same time we were there in the OR. I opened some discussion that helped them calm down and focus on keeping her organs as good as they could be for the babies whose lives we could save. Communication between the heart and lung teams was crucial as timing was essential with the donor and with the recipient, so multiple phone calls were being made by me and their TC's. In the meantime I was trying to make contact with the social worker who was supposed to be helping me with the family. She finally answered after the fifth page and in no uncertain terms told me that she would not help me after the recovery; she believed the TC before me who got consent did so in some unethical way, which was the furthest thing from the truth. The reality was she had worked for more than 24 hours to help this young mom find closure and allow her baby to live on in another human being. At that point it was my job to close that loop. I did manage to get the OR charge nurse to help me gather the family members into a room.

Back in the OR they were minutes away from cross clamp. The cardiac monitors were still beeping, perfusionists were moving quickly to get the preservation bags of fluid hung, primed and ready to go and basins of ice were waiting on the back table. The heart guy announced he was ready, anesthesia was silent, the large clamp was applied across the aorta just above the femoral arteries and the surgeon cut the aorta and vena cava. The sound of suctioning and tense orders from the surgeons calling for ice and for the perfusionist to turn on the flow overpowered the beeping monitor at first ... then, silence. The heart had stopped. The surgeon removed it from the chest, flushed it and examined it on the back table and began packaging it in ice. The lung doctors had already starting the process of removal and the lungs were out minutes after the heart. It was the same process: back table, flush with cold, sugary fluid, examination, pictures were obtained by the perfusionist and then off they went. I was making rapid phone calls to the office that was allocating the kidneys, to my boss and to the recipient surgeons with crucial information about timing, anatomy and status of the organs. I was also making phone calls to security for escorts out the nearest exit, to the ambulances waiting to leave for the plane and to the helicopter service to let them know they could get ready to fly. The OR staff was very quiet. I was actually thankful for how much I had to do right then because if I had stopped to think I might never have stopped crying. I tried to focus on the babies about to receive these precious gifts.

Once the surgeons had gone, the OR staff began the process of cleaning up. The surgical tech cleaned the baby up and suggested packing the baby's abdomen with lap sponges to give her some weight because the mom wanted to see her. She also suggested we wrap the baby in blankets from the warmer in case the mom wanted to touch her. I don't know how I would have gotten through that next hour without this one girl from the OR. She told me they had a viewing room up by the morgue because when children died in the OR parents frequently wanted to see them after death.

As we pushed her little bassinet through the back halls up to the morgue I stopped to check in with the morgue attendant before heading to the viewing room. I knew this was possibly going to be one of the hardest things I had ever done in my career in healthcare, but it was necessary. We took her into a small room with some chairs; the mom came in and had an outfit she wanted to dress her in, she even had little frilly socks to match. We unwrapped the blankets, and the mom reluctantly reached down to touch her. She tried to lift her tiny shoulders to slip the shirt on and the baby's head fell back and the mom lost it. She sat down and sobbed so we dressed the baby in the outfit and the other family members began to filter into the room. The maternal grandmother, who was 40, the same age as me, asked if she could hold her and I said of course. She walked over and gently picked the baby up out of the bassinette, held her to her face and sobbed, crying like she would never stop, knowing their lives would never be the same. The young mother just sat alone, silent in a chair in the corner. I was crying openly at this point, completely unable to prevent myself from being affected by their grieving. There were about 25 family members present and each one, with the exception of a few, held the baby. When they started leaving the room one by one, I was finally left alone with the mom. I gently placed the infant in her arms and she cradled her close to her body. I sat across from her in a chair, silent, crying, wondering how I could ever be the same after that experience, longing to go home and hold my own girls that were so full of life. I watched this young mother adjust the outfit she brought, smooth the baby's silky black hair with her hands and look down at her as if imprinting this image, this feeling of the baby in her arms into her mind forever. She finally spoke and said to me, "I'm sorry. I just can't let her go yet." I told her she could take all the time she needed even though inside I felt like I might not be able to stand the sadness of the situation for one more second. I watched her though, and could see that somewhere inside of herself she was looking for closure, for peace. It was only about 10 minutes later that she looked up at me; no more tears left in her, and said, "You can take her now." I tried to refrain from sobbing when she gently handed her to me. I placed her in the bassinette and turned to this brave young girl, I embraced her, crying, thanking her for the incredible gift she gave when she had no hope left, telling her I hoped this was the worst thing she would ever go through and that the rest of her life would be better. What could you say to someone in that situation?

The mom left and I took the baby to the morgue attendant. He commented that I looked as if I had been through "a war" and efficiently took her from me, tied the toe tag, put her in the miniature plastic body bag and placed her on a shelf in the fridge. I began the exhaustive walk to my car.

Following the procedure I called both the clinical phone coordinator and my Administrator on Call (AOC), and reported that I was finished, all went well, the viewing was over, the medical examiner was called and I was again available to be called somewhere else. I sat down on the bench that overlooked the main lobby of the children's hospital and felt so drained I wasn't sure I could drive myself home. Suddenly my Blackberry rang. It was my AOC. I thought, "oh no, not this soon," but instead of sending me elsewhere, he asked me, "Are you OK?" A simple question that caused an overflow of emotion, "not really," was my reply. He said, "Go home, take a hot shower and snuggle up next to your daughters. Don't worry about going out the rest of today. You need to recover." I thanked him in between sobs and drove home, the whole way thinking about the day. I came through my front door and as I did many times after dealing so closely with death, I grabbed both my daughters and held them close, crying. They would just say, "We love you mom. Tough case, huh?"

After I got settled, took a shower and got something to eat, I sat down in my pajamas to log into our active patient system (known as the "board," which many of us, including myself, stalked when on call to see what was going on with fellow TC's who were also on call). My Blackberry showed a blinking red light that meant I had a message or email. Sitting in my inbox was an email from the TC that had obtained consent from the mom and a message saying, "check this out" with a link. I clicked the link and a website instantly popped up about a three-year-old girl in North Carolina who had just received a lifesaving liver, pancreas and intestine transplant. My coworker had done something we rarely did, she Googled the recipient's name thinking it was a rare transplant and something might be in the news, leading her to that website. Adorable pictures of the little girl were all over the website, as well as a blog by her mother. I scrolled through her postings, which included many false alarms where they had rushed to the hospital, even having the baby taken to the OR only to have something go wrong in the end. Her postings also reflected the progression of her daughter's illness, and then there were postings from the previous two days. These postings included when they got the call, how they felt rushing to the hospital, how she grieved for the baby donor's mother, how she appreciated the selfless gift of life, each post ending with the line, "R.I.P. baby angel." I cried for most of the next two days on and off because even though I knew I was an integral part of saving the little girl's life, I also could not forget that another life that barely existed had been lost.

■

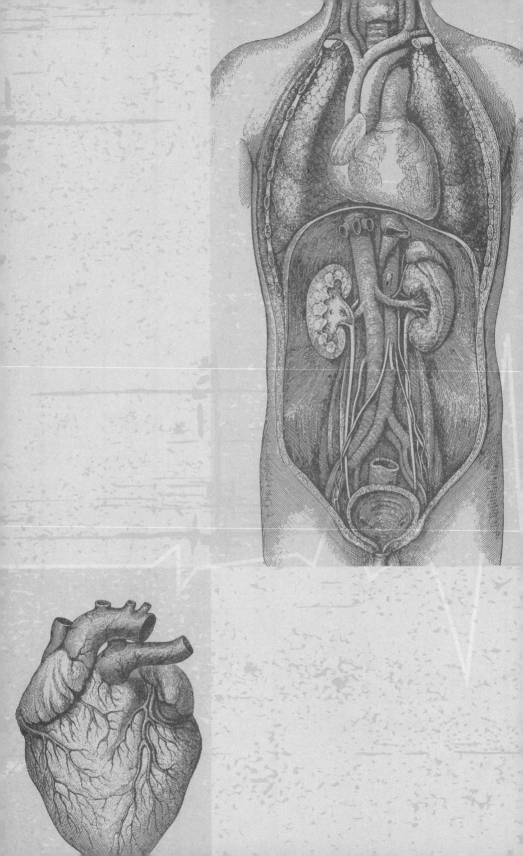

12

The Family Conversation

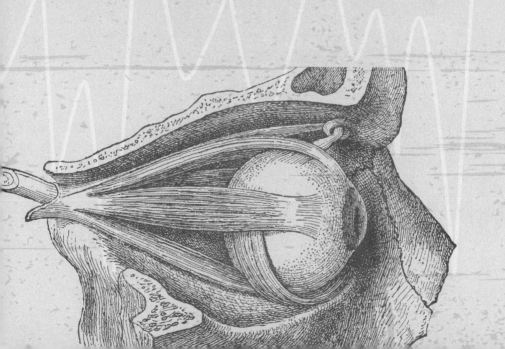

THE LYRICS TO JOHN MAYER'S SONG "SAY WHAT YOU NEED TO SAY" HAVE always reminded me of how it felt walking into the family conversation. "It's just a conversation" they used to say in consent training. I had them with many combinations of family members, sometimes just with a spouse and sometimes just with the children or parents of the donor. It didn't matter who was in the room, these were the hardest situations I'd ever been in and I remember every family I met with, all of them. We had extensive training in this process. Days and days of practice consent workshops every three months in which we spent the day in groups, role playing every possible scenario and objection the family could throw at you. To say these conversations are awkward is an understatement, yet it only takes one family, in their worst possible grief, to sit in front of you and say "yes" to change your life.

We were trained to sit through the uncomfortable silences and give quiet support while family members cried or expressed anger or frustration at the events that had led them there. People generally think of organ donors as young, healthy people who have suffered some kind of tragedy. In reality we evaluated people as old as 85 and as young as two months. They called this "casting a wide net" so as not to miss any opportunity. I have one of those magnet ribbons on my car that says, "organ donors save lives" and that is so true although many times the donors go unrecognized by the recipient. We considered ourselves to be dual advocates of both sides but we had much closer contact with the donors. It would be impossible for me to write this book and not speak for all the donor families. I have had the opportunity to have several organ recipients in my current career as a home health nurse. When I asked if they had written to the donor family, one said she did many years ago and the other said that she couldn't bring herself to write. One of my patients got her kidney from a young male, almost a perfect match, 12 years earlier. I told her that the family of that kid would love to know she was still alive 12 years later. She seemed to shrug it off and when I mentioned it to her daughter once she told me she felt the family wouldn't want to have "flashbacks" and if they wrote it could cause that to happen. I told her I strongly disagreed and as someone who had sat with many of these families I certainly felt confident that I was right. I encouraged my other patient to write to her donor family as well, even if it was just to say, "I don't know what to say except thank you." The donors had given selflessly at the worst times of their lives and it was always an honor to be a part of it. Most donor families truly believe their loved one will live on in another human being so why wouldn't they want to hear how that person is doing? Until I did home healthcare I really had no idea how bad it is for patients who are waiting for a kidney, getting dialysis three times a week for about five to seven hours. Some go in the middle of the night because they can stay on the machines longer and get better results. Firstly, they have to endure gaining access to even start dialysis, which means they have surgery to put a vein and artery together called an arteriovenous (AV) fistula because the catheter is too big to put in just one vein or artery. They can't use that for about three months so they also have catheters placed for the interim, usually in a large vein in the chest or neck. They have constant issues with blood pressure and electrolytes, some even are given bouillon cubes in hot water just to get their blood pressure high enough to get out of the chair. As a home health nurse nurse I have found that if you have an issue with the patient you have to call the dialysis clinic. The nurses there are knowledgeable but have an attitude sometimes, as if they are asking, "what else do you want me to do? We already are keeping him alive."

Talking about dialysis was an effective way of opening up conversation, especially if the family knew someone who is going through it. I now want to highlight some of the conversations I had, both ones that went well and ones that went badly.

Early in my training I was at one of the pediatric hospitals with another Transplant Coordinator who was training me. During a brutal part of training, 14 straight days on call rotation, you were sent everywhere with these senior TC's from the Organ Procurement Organization, called preceptors. Once I was on the pediatric Intensive Care Unit with a TC in her mid 20s and eight months pregnant with her first baby. The patient was a two-year-old who they believed had been accidently suffocated when the mother had rolled over onto her. The mother of the child was only 18 and unmarried, lived in the inner city and was uneducated. Pronouncing infants and toddlers brain dead takes longer than adults, usually 48 hours unless there is a very specific devastating injury, but they were ready to pronounce her. We first met with the mom, her mother and the paternal grandfather and tried to ascertain how much they understood about what was happening. Because I was in training I was more than happy to let my preceptor talk to them. I knew she was struggling internally. When the preceptor transitioned into talking about organ donation all hell broke loose. The young mom stood up and yelled that we were just trying to take her baby's organs and to get the "fuck" out of the room! The preceptor was in tears, I was shaken up, the nurse was upset and the mother was hysterical. Not the scene we liked to cause and of all days we had the hardest Administrator on Call, who insisted we "re-approach" her. I had been quiet up to that point but I felt I had nothing to lose so I said that I noticed when we were in there that my preceptor never looked at or talked directly to the mom. I had been a teenage mom and I knew that if I was in that mom's shoes I would have said, "Hey, this is my baby, you need to talk to me, not them." The preceptor agreed to let me talk to the mom, I think mainly because she simply could not face doing it herself. The hospital chaplain helped us get everyone back together. I knew I wouldn't have her attention for very long so I looked her right in the eyes and said I realized how hard this must be for her, that I had been a mom at 18 and knew that was hard enough all by itself. I definitely got through to her on that level but she was a perfect example of someone who didn't understand her daughter was dead and therefore the thought of donating her organs was unfathomable. The baby had no marks on her and looked like she was asleep. The nurse was helping the mom make a plaster handprint of the baby's little hand as we left the unit.

I had another very disturbing conversation with a Greek family in a city hospital. Their daughter was only 26 and she had been taking Percocet for a whiplash injury she sustained in a car accident. She had a headache one day, popped a couple Excedrins and went right into liver failure from the overdose of acetaminophen. In my two and a half years doing that job I saw five times as many patients overdose from prescription drugs than from heroin. She had spent three days at the top of the liver recipient list but unfortunately, if liver enzymes or ammonia (which the liver processes) get too high, they literally fry the brain. I was onsite before pronouncement, the girl was not donor designated on her driver's license but the doctors were getting ready to do the second exam. I sat and talked to the pretty female resident, who was herself Greek. She was going to be the one who would tell the family their daughter had died so I needed to brief her about what to say and what not to say. I told her to definitely tell them the time of death, explain that the time would not change when she came off the ventilator and make sure to use the words "died" or "dead," as harsh as they may seem. It didn't help the family to pretend, they deserved to know the truth, and it was up to us as healthcare professionals to bring them to an understanding of what had happened. I also told her not to mention anything about organ donation because it could be perceived as a conflict of interest by the family. "No problem" she said and walked down the hall. She came out of the family's room about 20 minutes later and said they were ready for me. She took me down to the room, introduced me as someone the hospital partners with in these situations and I sat down to talk to the parents, brother and uncle of this young girl. The uncle was more concerned with following the young resident out the door because he was pathetically throwing himself at her. Her parents were older, obviously they had their kids later in life. Her brother looked to be about a year or two younger, he spoke perfect English but her parents spoke with heavy accents. I quickly found out they knew almost nothing about what had happened. I spent a long time helping them understand that Excedrin and Percocet both have Tylenol or acetaminophen in them and even a little bit more than you should take could cause immediate liver failure. It's kind of like Russian roulette though, you could do that a hundred times and have no problem but the next time, like this girl, it could kill you. When I said that the girl had been pronounced dead and told them the time of death everyone freaked out. The resident had not told them, which not the first or last time I was in that predicament. Her brother kept saying over and over, "No she's not dead, I will not accept that as her time of death." Again I had to explain that it's like your time of birth — once it's there, it never changes. So I transitioned by talking about how horrible it was that she couldn't get a liver and how rare organ donors actually were, then I asked if they understood that their daughter was a potential organ donor. They were upset but said that she would not have wanted that and that she had insisted her father and brother take the designation off their own licenses. I talked about how they felt waiting to see if a match would come and how many people there were in the same boat, some of them in that same hospital. It didn't matter what I said, they kept refusing to consider the idea.

At one point this grieving family even tried to tell me that if the patient herself had known her only chance for survival was a liver transplant she would have refused. Figuring I had nothing to lose I said, "So let me get this straight, you were fine waiting for someone else to die and donate a liver to your daughter, but now you don't want her to be a donor?" Yes, they all said. I ended it politely by saying, "This has gone in the wrong direction, I think this conversation is over" and left the room, sending the resident back in to deal with the aftermath — she deserved it. The nurses on that ICU were not happy with that family's decision but I always defended the family, whatever they chose to do. I don't know that I could donate one of my kid's organs so I never judge others. My AOC, of course, was pissed and instructed me to, "stay there until she's in the body bag" in case they change their minds. The resident came out and asked how long the family could stay with her, her nurse replied, "One hour, then she's going to the morgue." I stayed and they didn't change their minds. The nurse said to me, "what a waste" as she zipped up the bag on the morgue cart. I agreed.

I was called to another inner-city hospital once where there was a very large African American family present for the donor. He only had one child though, a daughter, and she was on her way, but so was his ex-wife, the daughter's mother. I first met with the daughter once the doctors were finished talking to her, but it wasn't long before we were surrounded by the other family members. The mother claimed to be an ordained minister and walked around as if she was royalty. She dominated every conversation, except the one I was in charge of. I spoke directly to the daughter, explaining brain death and what it meant. Her mother, like a devil on her shoulder, kept saying god would bring a miracle, once the tube was removed he would breathe. I told her daughter the sad truth, he had already been pronounced clinically brain dead; once the tube was removed he would not breathe and his heart would stop, but at that point it would be too late for donation of his liver or kidneys. I told her that her father still had a healthy liver and kidneys and I could tell his daughter wanted to do the right thing and say yes, but was definitely concerned with the backlash from her mother. I ended up having to hold the consent conversation with the entire family, maybe 15 people in all. The medical-social questionnaire we gave every donor had some very personal questions about sexual behavior or if the donor had ever been in prison. This family answered yes, he had been in prison, but refused to say for what, not that it mattered. I've had family members get very upset when I ask if their loved ones ever exchanged sex for money or drugs, or if they ever used recreational drugs. But it is important for the safety of the recipients. Before they all left the mother asked for my number so she could invite me to her prayer meetings because she felt I needed a prayer. What really mattered in the end was that her father saved three lives with the donation of his liver and two kidneys that day.

I went to a referral not long after I had finished my training where I needed to go in and speak with the family as soon as I arrived at the hospital. They were waiting to withdraw life support and the nurse had run out of excuses for stalling. I arrived just in time and gathered the family in a room. I started the conversation by telling them how I was trained and finding out what they knew when one of the women said, "Who are you?" I hesitated for a minute, I really hated that we were taught to be vague about who we were, so she said it again a little more emphatically, "Who are you? Why are you here?" I decided to just say it, "I'm from the Organ Donor Program." There, the cat was out of the bag. One of the women was a retired charge nurse from that very same hospital and had worked with us in the past, the other one questioning me was a local paramedic. They all relaxed a bit at that point and some were even chuckling a little. I asked the patient's daughter if she thought her mother would have wanted to help save two or three lives through the donation of her kidneys and liver. They all told me in no uncertain terms that the patient was the "most selfish person" they all knew and wouldn't give anything to anyone. I truly did not know what to say. This was one of those situations where it didn't really matter, her organs probably were not transplantable anyway, but the OPO believed emphatically that every family deserved the opportunity to make the choice to at least evaluate. I thanked them for their honesty and hit the road.

Sometimes when uncomfortable family situations needed to be discussed you got blindsided by really unexpected obstacles. I was referred to a 54-year-old man in the city and met with his four sisters and his mother to discuss donation after cardiac death. Part of having to get consent is ensuring you are asking the right people. Everyone these days loves to say they have "power of attorney." We had to follow a strict hierarchy though, regardless of who had power of attorney, if there was a spouse, estranged or not, they came first. I will also add that most power of attorneys are null and void once a patient is pronounced brain dead, which this patient was not. If there was no spouse, next of kin would be the children, then siblings except when a parent was still alive in which case they would be next of kin over a sibling.

I was in the middle of the medical-social questionnaire with the family when one sister answered yes to the question of whether the father had ever been in prison. Another sister told me the patient had 10 biological children ranging in age from 18 to 30. I thought, oh great, I've done all this work and now I'm going to have to talk to the oldest child. The sisters were looking at each other and I could tell something else was coming. Finally, one of them said he had been in prison because he was accused of molesting all 10 kids. I can't recall how I moved the conversation along from there because it was like a blur, all I could think about was that my AOC was not going to be happy. I wrote down everyone's cell phone numbers and promised to be in touch later with a plan. We were still in the waiting phase of the process. I went back to the nurse's station and made the dreaded call to my AOC to review the medical-social questionnaire and when I came to the part about why he was in prison he immediately said, "You need to find them."

I knew he was going to say that, damn it. I started trying to call his sisters and got no answer from the first one. Second one, no answer. The third one answered, I asked if she knew where the kids were or how to contact them. She said she may be able to get in touch with the youngest one and asked why I needed to talk to her. I explained that legally the children were this man's next of kin when it came to consent for donation and that we didn't follow the same hierarchy as the hospital. Then she told me the best thing I had heard all day, the patient had given up all parental rights as the father when he was in prison. Problem solved and a narrowly escaped horrific situation for me.

Thankfully, the good conversations far outweighed the bad ones and that includes some that did not result in donation. I have shared some unforgettable moments with some of these families. On many occasions, completing the medical-social questionnaire became a time of memories and I laughed and cried with the families while they shared details about their loved ones. I remember in particular one conversation about an elderly woman who drowned while swimming in the ocean, one of the things she most liked to do. I met with her three adult children, they knew their mother's wish was to be a donor if she was ever in the position and now that time had come. One of the questions on the medical-social questionnaire asked if the donor had any digestive problems. Her kids all looked at each other, sitting all on one couch, and the two older ones looked at the youngest with that, "don't you dare say it" look. Too late. She spoke up and told me that her mom had the worst gas of anyone she had ever known and was constantly "farting loudly." She said to her siblings, "Come on, you know she did." It actually turned into a funny moment and I really bonded with that family, although I didn't mention that I was praying my kids would never admit to anything that embarrassing about me! Some families enjoyed the questions because it gave them a break from the grief—talking about the donor's life, not their death.

I had a donor just three days after Christmas. The patient had experienced a massive stroke at home in front of his children on Christmas day. His wife was also a Registered Nurse and they had seven adopted children ranging in age from their early 20s to just four years old. All had witnessed their father lighting a fire and then collapsing right in front of the fireplace. All of them came into the hospital that night to say their goodbyes. Once the kids came and spent some time with him his wife sent them all home, she wanted to stay until he went to the OR. We evaluated all his organs but it looked as if only the liver and kidneys were possible and his liver had a high potential for being declined because he was overweight. If the liver is too fatty it can't be used; a fatty liver puts the recipient at risk for a fat emboli or a globule of fat that gets into the artery and heads to the heart or brain, causing death. We even did a cardiac catheterization in hopes we could place his heart but it just wasn't going to work. So I moved ahead, scheduling the OR and getting transportation for the teams.

At that point it was 3 a.m. and I went looking for his wife to update her. It was snowing outside and I found her sitting alone in a dark waiting room outside the unit. She was watching the snow silently fall through a large window. I sat down next to her, a fellow nurse, I didn't know what else to do for her. As I sat next to her in silence watching the snow fall she said, "I want to show you something." She pulled out her phone and tapped on the camera icon, which brought up a video. After she hit play she leaned toward me so I could see. There was her husband playing with their four-year-old son on the bed, both of them laughing hysterically while they roughhoused. She said she had recorded it just a day before the stroke. We watched it several times, both crying, and then she dialed into her voicemail. There was a message from her husband, just checking in with her, seeing how her day went, he said, "Love ya, see you at home." She looked at me and said, "That's all I have left of him." She made me understand deeply how you never know when it may be the last time you see or talk to someone.

She said she usually deleted all his voicemails but had missed that one. I will never forget how I felt sitting there with her in the dark. I have never appreciated my husband more than at that moment. I try very hard to live my life knowing that anytime you leave someone or even just go to sleep, it could be the last time. You simply never know.

The ability of these families to say yes when all hope for their loved one was lost was nothing short of amazing. Many said they didn't want someone else to suffer like they suffered. Our OPO honored these donor families in an annual ceremony that was always very emotional but beautifully done. Families were invited after the first year anniversary of the death and were encouraged to send in pictures and make a quilt square about their loved one. People made incredibly personalized quilt squares, we sent them fabric and some ideas and all the little pieces were sewn together in large display quilts. Many of our hospital partners proudly displayed them in their lobbies. I found that a common denominator in all of these families was they didn't want their loved one to be forgotten, ever. Organ donors are heroes that save lives and heroes are never forgotten.

■

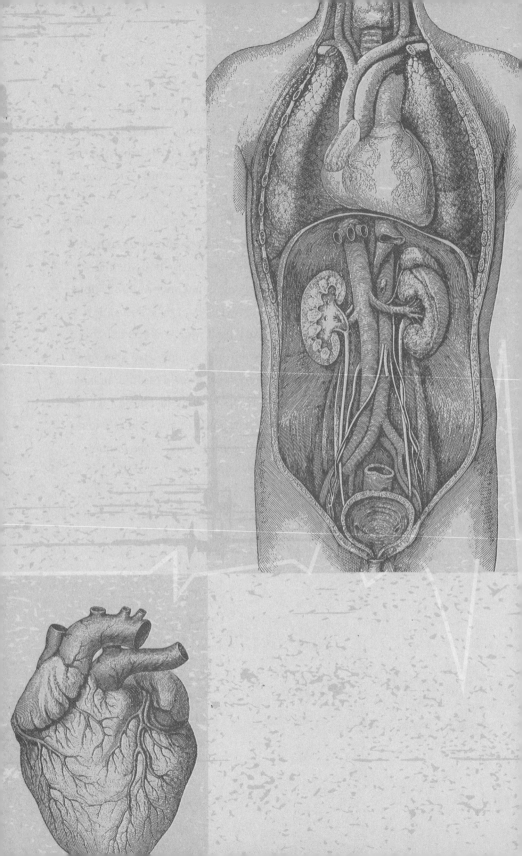

13

The Heart

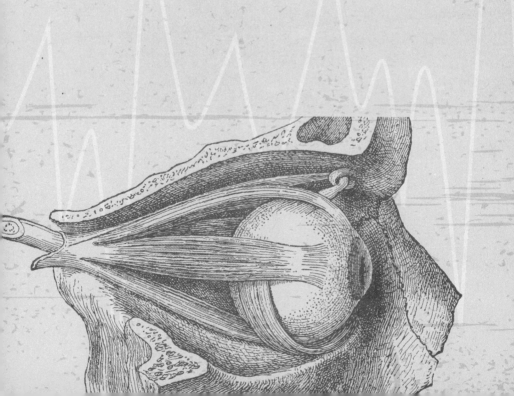

O UT OF ALL THE ORGANS THAT CAN BE TRANSPLANTED, THE HEART seems to have the most meaning to donor families. Unfortunately it's not that common to get a heart transplanted. As Transplant Coordinators we all lived and worked by the mantra "every organ, every time." It was drilled into us. We would try very hard to get a donor heart in good enough shape to transplant. The fact that there are mile radius limits on all thoracic organs means that if someone you know got a heart, it came from relatively close by. The heart and lungs can only be outside of the body for four hours and that includes travel time.

I've had a few memorable experiences involving the heart that seem to indicate that there is a mystery surrounding this organ that is not found with any other. There are stories about heart transplant patients having aversions or cravings for things after surgery that they didn't have before the transplant. I've done some research on this subject and know that human cells have a memory — some people believe that is the answer to the mystery of the new cravings. Makes sense to me.

One of my early cases involved a young man, 21 years old, who had been taking a type of anabolic steroid to bulk up for college football. His friends told me late in the night as they sat vigil at his bedside that he had never wanted to work out, he just wanted to be big. He had been feeling like he had the flu for a couple days and had some abdominal pain. His friend took him to the local Emergency Room and he was immediately transferred into a city hospital and was listed as a potential liver recipient. He was a typical, healthy 21-year-old enjoying college and was very popular judging by the number of students who came to see him. I believe the entire girls soccer team came. It was about 24 hours after admission when the doctors realized that his ammonia level had become so elevated that it had literally cooked his brain. One of the many functions of the liver is to process and metabolize ammonia, his liver had shut down and ceased to do this. The boy's father was completely devastated. I had my first consent conversation with his dad without another TC present. It was very touching when his father showed extreme pride when I told him his son had chosen to be an organ donor on his driver's license. I cried with him and told him that my own son was the same age. I remember after the conversation I told a TC who was training me that I had broken down when I spoke to the father and his response was, "As long as it was sincere." I thought that was a strange thing to say, but I blew it off. I was there most of the night, as were his friends. His father went home, saying he would return in the morning with his other son who was a Marine. From what I was told the brother had been on his way overseas and was flown back to the U.S. by the American Red Cross due to his only brother's death.

The young man's friends sat outside his Intensive Care Unit (ICU) room all night, sharing funny stories with me and the hospital staff about their buddy. I have to give credit to the ICU staff at this hospital; not once did anyone limit the amount of visitors or the number of times they came. They understood what a sad situation it was. The ICU charge nurse even brought in two dozen donuts in the morning for the staff and family. I honestly think he wasn't even scheduled to work that day.

The next day the father and brother showed up early. Neither one had slept and it showed. His brother pulled me aside in the hallway and while ·standing right next to a "Donate Life" poster asked me to bring him up to speed on what had happened. I remember he was a tall, very handsome, clean-cut young man. When I told him everything he did not show any emotion at all. I told him it was OK if he needed to break down or get angry and his reply was, "I'm a U.S. Marine, I was trained not to show my emotions." One very important thing I learned doing this job was never, ever judge someone based on how they deal with death. There is no right or wrong way to do it and everyone will deal with it in time, no matter how they try not to think about it. He knew that I had been a source of comfort and support for his grieving father and was grateful. They stayed with the patient as we got things ready to head to the Operating Room (OR) and even the usually hurried OR staff did not push to get moving, everyone allowed them time to say a final goodbye. It was heart wrenching.

This young man ended up being a full donor except for his liver; five lives were saved and many others enhanced by tissue donation. There was some drama in the OR when the kidney surgeon made an extra incision that he didn't have permission to do and the TC with me freaked out. The surgeon had made a very small incision across the mid-abdomen to have better access to the kidney. Once closed it would not be noticeable at all, but the rules were the rules. He knew he was in trouble when his senior partner showed up, in fact his exact words were, "Uh oh, am I done doing donors?" He apologized and I'm sure he got a talking to afterward, but they needed him so he wasn't done doing anything. I had told the young man's brother and father that I would call them when we were done with the organ recovery, which would probably not be before 4 p.m. that afternoon. They were meeting with a funeral director that day to start arrangements and didn't want to miss my call. The strange thing was around 2:30 p.m. my Blackberry rang and I recognized the brother's number. I answered but asked him to hold on a second. When I came back to the phone his brother informed me he knew it was early but he had a very strong urge to call me. I was a little stunned and told him that actually, just as he had called, the heart surgeon was walking out the door of the OR with his brother's heart. Neither one of us really knew what to say but I heard his brother give a little chuckle, like he wasn't surprised. I stayed in touch with his father until I saw him at the donor ceremony a year and a half later. He had been struggling the entire time but when he came he had a quilt patch the family had made in honor of the young man and proudly brought it up to the big piece of fabric hanging in front of the room just as a large picture appeared on the digital screen of his son. We had a talk about writing to the recipients while we had coffee afterward and I encouraged him to try. He told me he felt different after the ceremony, that he had obtained a kind of closure and felt he absolutely would write to all of them.

I was the TC on a case in one of the big city hospitals where we were only able to transplant the heart of a beautiful young female who had battled with alcoholism for most of her adult life. She was another donor whose elevated liver enzymes caused brain damage and it was a really challenging case. When I arrived on the ICU and walked into her room I was shocked by what I saw. There was this tiny, emaciated patient, dark brown in color from her liver failure, and she had an old-fashioned football helmet on her head. She had suffered from a complication of her alcoholism where, secondary to the liver damage, the portal vein in her liver got kind of backed up, called portal hypertension, and it caused the veins in her esophagus to become very dilated, like varicose veins in the esophagus. They are called esophageal varices and if they rupture they bleed profusely. Usually once that happens the healthcare team will make last-ditch efforts to stop the bleeding using something called a Blakemore tube. It is basically a tube that goes in the esophagus and has a large area of foam around itself to tamponade the bleeding veins. Tamponade means to apply direct pressure to a bleeding area, but from the inside. For this patient, in order to hold the Blakemore tube in place they secured it with the football helmet because the pressure from the veins was so strong it could have pushed the tube out. Her eyes were literally bulging out of her head to the point that her eyelids could no longer cover them and they were very yellow from jaundice. She had received many units of blood and her kidneys had shut down after her liver. Believe it or not though, her heart was healthy. Patients of a certain age and smoking history require a cardiac catheterization to look at the major coronary arteries under an X-ray before determining if the heart is transplantable. Any blockages are easily visible. We would sometimes work all night if the heart had some acute damage or dysfunction, using a drug called Dobutamine in a drip. It was like exercising the donor's heart to see how well it could function. All heart donors required an ultrasound of the heart, called an echocardiogram, and the TC had to ensure the tech made a CD for the recipient team. This was usually a problem in the middle of the night because the cardiology residents could work the ultrasound machine but could not burn a CD. This young lady's husband gave consent for donation and we moved forward, ruling out most of the organs based on her current condition. It looked as if the heart was going to be the only organ we could use and it was going to someone at the same hospital.

Pronouncement had been a challenge due to her elevated liver enzymes and required many, many conversations with the unit's medical director. I don't know why she was on a pulmonary ICU but she was and I had to work around it. The pulmonologist who was going to be the pronouncing physician was not used to doing brain death exams, especially when you had problems like the inability to certify that the patient's electrolytes were within normal limits. The doctors continued to look up policies and tried to make a decision while my Administrator on Call (AOC) continued to push me, saying that someone's life was at stake so we'd better figure it out. Many times the attending surgeon asked me why we had to do the brain death exams, couldn't we just let her go? These exams were often the more difficult and time-consuming course of action, for the family and the hospital. So when he would start to complain I would say, "I don't know, how about you walk over to the cardiac ICU and take a look to see how sick the recipient is?" Of course, I was being a smartass but this went on between us for hours.

Finally I went over and sat down next to him as he continued to frantically search the online policy and procedure manual and said, "I know brain death pronouncement can be done, I have seen it done on other units and other hospitals. The last time was here on the trauma/neuro ICU, let's see who is working tonight." We called over to the ICU and the night attending was a trauma fellow who couldn't really help so we made the decision to reach out in the middle of the night to one of the doctors who frequently worked with us. He called us back within two minutes and the attending with me explained the situation — basically he had no idea how to get around the certification that her electrolytes were within normal limits, which he would need to do for brain death pronouncement. With her liver and kidney failure her sodium was high and we were having trouble regulating fluids and potassium. The trauma doctor knew what to do though and after a lengthy discussion between them, including the need for updating the brain death policy for these situations. Whew, that only took 16 hours. Her husband had given me a picture of the girl taken before she got sick and she was beautiful. I promised him I would make sure everyone who took care of her saw the picture; at this point she looked terrible.

The patient started to become unstable after about 22 hours of work and only an hour before our scheduled OR time. I called my AOC to tell him we were having problems and he asked if I was ready to go to the OR. Once I said yes, he said, "page your surgeon and go." We called the OR and alerted them that we were coming down and she was starting to become unstable. I knew if we could at least get to the Operating Room we would be OK, the anesthesia would stabilize her and if they couldn't stabilize her we would move to get the heart out immediately. Some of the nurses working with me also took care of the recipient so they wanted this to happen and boy did they show it. Once I told them the OR was ready they packed up all her lines and bagged her with what's called an ambu-bag that mimics the ventilator in an emergency. I gave the direction to open all IV lines wide to help keep her blood pressure up so we could get down there without her coding. The nurses at that point ran, literally ran down the hall, into the elevator, and again off the elevator all the way into the operating room. It was unbelievable to see, it was like you were watching a movie. As I had promised, I made sure everyone saw her picture in the OR. The anesthesia staff stabilized her and her healthy heart was transplanted in about two hours. I saw the surgeon involved the next day and he told me the recipient was already off the ventilator and eating.

Another experience that was a bit disturbing involved a brain-dead patient in her late 70s. She was a patient who had been taking Coumadin or blood thinners for atrial fibrillation. When she suddenly stopped taking them for some unknown reason, blood clots flowed all over her body including her brain. Her lab results showed she was constantly acidotic (too much acid in the blood) and she had bloody diarrhea that told me she had what we called a dead bowel. This condition produced a very distinct rotting fish smell. I had encountered it many times in my days in the OR. Stopping the blood thinners threw bloodclots to her internal mesenteric arteries that supplied the colon and intestines with blood. When the bowel dies or becomes necrotic it happens fast, is irreversible unless resected and sends so many toxins into the blood stream that the organs cannot be transplanted. Despite all this my AOC was not budging, he said there was no definitive test for dead bowel and that the family wanted to try to make something good come out of her death. So we would do just that — try. I scheduled the OR time and arranged for the surgeon to come and recover the liver and kidneys. Of course once he made the incision he knew that she had dead bowel, about 25 feet of it, so nothing was used for transplant but the family donated a lung to research.

The patient had had pulmonary fibrosis and little is known about it. In order to get to the lung they needed to remove her heart temporarily. They cut the big vessels and passed it into the hands of the surgical tech who turned around, stunned by the fact that it was beating in his hands. He gently placed it on his back table and the heart continued to beat with no blood in it for about seven minutes. I know because I watched the clock; the room was silent except for an occasional remark of disbelief from one of the OR staff. This patient was supposedly brain dead and that meant her heart should have stopped as soon as her oxygen was stopped but it didn't. I had no explanation, everyone was looking at me and I didn't know what to say. I talked to my AOC about it the next day and she said, "Are you sure she was dead?" I said, "I sure hope so, we took her to the Operating Room and cut her open." One of the very worst situations I had to face was to call a family that wanted to make a donation and tell them nothing was useable because of some problem. That whole case kind of made me feel sick to my stomach.

The allocation process for thoracic organs was always very exciting. It was done in an exact, consistent manner using a computerized national list of recipients, matched by blood type for everything but the heart and kidneys, they needed to be matched by human leukocytic antigen (HLA) cells. Think of the HLA cells as a mini defense system for our kidneys and heart to protect them from intruders or infection. But if the patient's HLA cells do not match at least four of the six HLA cells from the donor (we all have six HLA types on our kidneys), the patient's body will reject the donated organ. In severe cases of mismatching the heart can be rejected on the operating room table, thankfully this rarely happens. There was a nationally reported case about a little girl getting a mismatched heart and lungs years ago; she rejected the heart instantly and they tried to get another but were unsuccessful.

Once you had your list of potential recipients by blood type and HLA, you started calling surgeons at any time of day or night, no answering services or multiple-choice options, calls were made directly to the recipient surgeons' cell phones. I would say, "Hello Dr. so and so, this is Traci from the Organ Donor Program. I'm at such and such hospital with a 52-year-old male, closed-head injury, pronounced at 2:14 a.m. this morning. Your patient is at the top of the list, looking to go to the Operating Room around 8 a.m." They would usually ask a few questions about who was next on the list overall and who was next for them. Since I was in an area that had many transplant centers, sometimes there were multiple patients from the same center listed and the surgeons always wanted to know if they had more than one patient coming up. We would give them some recent lab results, the results of the cardiac catheterization if it had been done and the echo (ultrasound of the heart) results. They would call back a few minutes later to let you know if they were accepting. If they declined, a code popped up on the list that correlated to a reason, like "donor quality" or "recipient is too sick for transplant." The heart and lung lists did not have the sickest waiting recipients on them because surgeons would not transplant a heart into a patient if it was questionable that they would survive post-operation. They also did what we called "pull other organs," for example if a recipient was number one or two on the heart list and was also on the liver or kidney list, no matter where they were on that liver or kidney list, they would get those organs too.

If the surgeon accepted the organs, you set the OR time with the heart surgeon and everything else had to follow. You arranged transportation to and from if needed, sometimes we would even put a plane on standby at the airport just in case they got the chance to come as one of the backups. It was a rare opportunity for heart or lungs to be transplanted and everyone in the field knew it.

I worked with a woman once whose son, a U.S. Marine, had died in a tragic accident. He came to the aid of a girl who was being bullied by her boyfriend. He was punched in the chin, fell back and hit his head on the curb, causing a fatal brain injury. The family donated his organs and the mother even met the heart recipient. When the recipient died she was devastated, explaining that in some strange way it was like losing her son again.

■

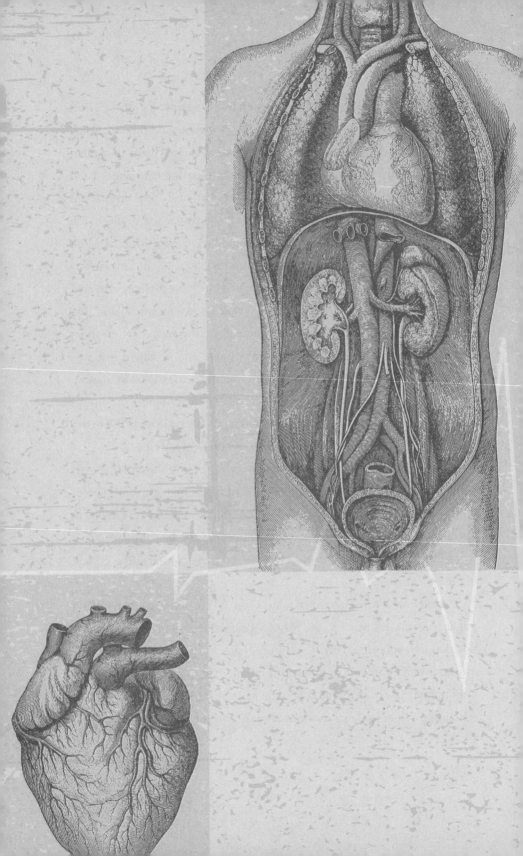

14

A Champion in Life and Death

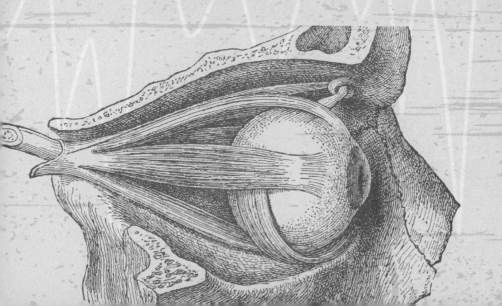

IT WAS NOVEMBER, A FEW DAYS BEFORE THANKSGIVING. I WAS ON CALL and just as I got out of the shower my pager went off. Great, it was only the first day of a 48-hour shift. I called back the number on my pager and spoke to one of my coworkers, a fellow Transplant Coordinator. She told me she had been at one of the city hospitals since about 1 a.m. the morning before getting consent for a young donor and I was her relief. I said I would call her when I was on the road and she could fill me in on the details. I finished getting dressed, packed my bags, kissed my girls and headed out the door. Once in the car I called my Administrator on Call to let them know I was on my way and then I called the person I was relieving. She would have enough time to give me the report 20 times, considering how long I spent in traffic. All I knew at that point was that she had gotten consent — that was a major thing I wouldn't have to do.

She started by telling me that the donor was a boxer who was there for a fight, collapsed in the 10th round and was pronounced the night before. "He's 25 and in perfect physical condition," she said. She had a lot to do dealing with the medical examiner so I told her when I thought I'd be arriving and said she could tell me the rest later.

I got to the hospital, parked on the roof and walked in to find two of my coworkers, the one I was relieving and an Advanced Practice Coordinator (APC), who was a TC with lots of experience. He was there to help make sure things ran smoothly. There is so much at stake with a young donor that you take all the help you can get. The TC started giving us the report, a healthy 25-year-old Latino male was in a boxing match at a nearby club and was hit a couple times in the first few rounds. He was a little woozy but he recovered and kept fighting because this was an important match for him. By the 10th round the fight was stopped because he was becoming unsteady, he sat down in his corner and complained of feeling very sleepy. He then collapsed on the mat and Emergency Medical Services (EMS) were called. The paramedics said he had no reflexes and appeared to be brain dead from the minute they got there. It was all so sad. Even though we all knew we had a very important job to do at that point, you could feel the sadness in everything we did and said. It hung over us like a fog that wouldn't go away.

The exhausted TC I was relieving, with huge dark circles under her eyes, filled us in on the details about pronouncement and how the family conversation went. The trauma director wanted to just tell them he was dead and move on, but the TC insisted he tell them slowly, so they could have time to process what had happened. The patient's young wife had just arrived from the airport when he was being pronounced. Other than being on the ventilator and having central IV lines, he looked like he was sleeping. The TC also insisted on having a priest there when she talked with this broken-hearted family. The man was the pride of his brothers and father, adored by his wife and mother and a loving, generous father to their year-old daughter. The family didn't want his body to go to waste, they understood the concept of him being a hero to the people he would save and they believed he would live on in the recipients. We did the physical assessment that was standard for all donors. He had several tattoos, some braided rope bracelets around his ankle and a prayer card written in Spanish in his right hand. She showed me that inside the card his wife had written "Te amo," meaning "I love you," and I promised I would make sure it stayed with him in the Operating Room.

After giving us the family contact information for the post-operation call, the TC left, emotionally and physically drained, to go home and sleep in case she was needed again later that night. I had never seen that TC so affected by a case; she was a tough little trauma nurse who had actually worked in that very same trauma Intensive Care Unit. She knew that she had given this family a way for their son to live on, but you could see the conflicting sadness we all felt at times as she stood silently over the patient and said a quiet goodbye. To this day she still wears a red, rhinestone-covered bead on a bracelet that reminds her of him and the passionate way he led his life.

Before we could begin allocating his organs we needed to have some critical tests completed and reported so the recipient surgeons could make an informed decision. We knew allocation would be easy because all his organs were in excellent condition. During the consent process the family had mentioned that they had an uncle who was waiting for a kidney transplant. The TC got the uncle's name, the transplant program where he was listed and his date of birth. She told them we would contact the uncle's surgeon to see if they were a match. We ordered an echocardiogram and a bronchoscopy. The echocardiogram would tell us how well his heart was functioning and the bronchoscopy would tell us if there were any abnormalities or infections in his lungs. The results turned out exactly as we had expected, excellent. His liver had the usual spike in enzymes over the first 24 hours from the trauma and blood loss in his head, but he was trending back down and that was what the liver surgeons wanted to see. It took more than 16 hours to accomplish all this work. Ten tissue packs, each containing five tubes of blood, were sent out via courier to local transplant centers for matching. We needed to make sure we had a copy on CD of the echocardiogram for the heart team and a report from the pulmonologist from the bronchoscopy, plus a recent chest X-ray to go with the lung team.

We knew that once we "hit the button" as we liked to call it, things would start to pick up speed. Hitting the button was what we called the start of allocating because you clicked on an icon on the National Organ Donor Network and it automatically notified multiple transplant surgeons simultaneously. We had the results of the most recent tests typed into his donor profile — lab tests to measure kidney function called Blood Urea Nitrogen (BUN) and creatinine; tests to measure liver function called Aspartate transaminase (AST), Alanine transaminase (ALT) and bilirubin; tests to check levels of cardiac enzymes to see if the heart was stressed and double checks on blood typing, one from the hospital lab and one from an independent lab. Serological testing was done to show if the donor had Hepatitis or HIV and arterial blood gases testing measured lung function and oxygen exchange. The results of all these tests were constantly updated in the file as they were received.

While we were waiting for the test results to come in we had a short break, so we grabbed a snack and some diet soda for the caffeine. When we got back I took my laptop and a chair into the patient's ICU room and set the laptop up on the windowsill. It was raining and windy outside, not a good night for flying. The APC who was with me felt we could allocate the heart, lungs and liver all at once so I opened up each list, told the site how many centers I wanted to notify and hit the button. I sat back and watched as each line changed from a little clock to a "notified" message. We waited a few minutes while we scanned each list. There was a heart recipient at the very top of the list in this same hospital. That would certainly make things easier. I decided to start making my calls. Starting at the top of the list I called the first heart surgeon, who answered on first ring. I said, "Hello, this is Traci from the Organ Donor Program. I see you have a provisional yes in for the heart." He told me he was accepting it and was very excited for his patient, a young 24-year-old right down the hall. I said I would let him know when I had an OR time. He said he would be waiting for my call. Next I called the lung surgeon at the top of the list who had another 24-year-old female recipient in the area. He also accepted immediately and wanted to know when I planned on heading to the OR. I told him I still had to place the liver and that the heart recipient was in this hospital so I would let him know. The room was very quiet, only the heart monitor beeping could be heard. I walked out to the nurse's desk to fax some results to the Organ Procurement Organization office that had people trained to allocate the kidneys, which was a very complicated procedure. The lists were thousands of people long and we would sometimes go to the OR knowing we had 48 hours to get the kidneys into a recipient. I was then approached by a young woman in a white lab coat and green scrubs, she introduced herself as one of the cardiology fellows taking care of the recipient. She told me how thrilled the team was that the family had graciously agreed to donate their son's organs, she told me how sick the young girl had been while waiting for a heart. She had just recently become critically ill and had been in the hospital for months, battling with her emotions, knowing that someone had to die to save her life yet hanging on to every day hoping, praying a heart would come. The doctor told me while choking back tears that they all thought she was going to die before getting a heart. "Not tonight," I thought to myself, "tonight she will receive the heart of a champion and her life will be saved." The liver recipient at the top of the list was a 25-year-old female, who must have been very sick. Patients waiting at the top of the liver list are sometimes only days from death. I called the surgeon, who accepted the liver immediately just like the others. They all knew how fortunate their patients were because of the gift this family had given. I was concerned about the liver team's transportation because of the wind and rain, but the surgeon told me, "Don't worry, we will just bring the big helicopter." I stopped for a minute to think about the significance of the ages and sexes of these three recipients, all around the patient's wife's age. I could only hope his wife could find some comfort in knowing he was saving their lives, pulling each one literally back from the brink of death, throwing them each a rope at the edge of the cliff.

I spoke with the OR charge nurse and the on-call anesthesiologist about setting a time so I could get the teams there. Our time was 1:30 a.m. I called our office, they would notify the perfusionist and arrange transportation for the lung team. My heart team was in house, my liver team was getting ready to fly and a limo was picking up the kidney and pancreas surgeon.

We changed into scrubs, packed our bags and made copies of the chart for each team. We could hear the thumping of a very large helicopter — the liver team was here. Once we knew all the teams were there we headed to the OR like a solemn procession through the halls. This was a pretty well-publicized case in the media and hospital staff on the floor knew who the donor was and where we were going. In the OR the circulating nurse and surgical tech were counting their instruments and our perfusionist was preparing her bags of fluid. The perfusionist came with large coolers of frozen sterile preservation solution. It was a sugary fluid used to flush the donor's vascular system as well as each organ on the surgical back table. The blood had to be washed out as soon as possible because even with the patient getting a very large dose of heparin (blood thinner) the blood could still clot within the organ. The perfusionist also smashed the frozen bags with a hammer and made sterile slush to dump into the abdomen. There were certain parts of the donor chart that needed to be reviewed with each surgeon before we could start. They had to review the pronouncement and death note by the pronouncing physician, the medical-social questionnaire, the serological testing for infectious diseases and the blood type. Then they had to each sign another document that verified they had reviewed those documents. As I started this process my coworker went into the OR to ensure that anesthesia didn't overload the heart and lungs with IV fluids, and that the patient had been given the required medications like mannitol, which helped the liver remain firm.

Many brain-dead donors have trouble regulating their fluids and electrolytes, only one of the hundred challenges in keeping a donor stable.

High sodium can cause what is called a "boggy liver," making the liver appear swollen, round and soft. A healthy liver has sharp, defined edges and a firm, smooth texture. If a boggy, sodium-soaked liver is transplanted the recipient can have problems regulating their sodium levels. Too much or too little sodium can be responsible for everything from edema to decreased reflexes. Mannitol is the first drug given once you are in the OR, followed by a paralytic, but brain-dead donors are not given any other sedation. As I was making sure that I had all the signatures I needed, my coworker came out to the hall and slipped something into my hand. I looked down and it was the prayer card. He said, "hold onto that so nothing happens to it." I slid it into my back pocket and walked into the OR.

The heart team led the way and was busy prepping and draping the patient. My coworker spoke up and said we would like to have a moment of silence out of respect for the donor. The emotion was palpable. After a few minutes the heart surgeon said he was ready to get started. The circulating nurse said the patient's name and that we were doing a multi-organ recovery; this was done in every OR across the country to prevent doing surgery on the wrong patient. An incision was made and the heart and lung teams worked in unison. There was constant communication between the teams working on the recipients. The liver team was very anxious, it seemed the recipient might have been a little unstable. As they continued dissecting as much as they could without cutting the aorta, they each talked a little about their recipients. The young girl getting the liver had a disorder that caused her to grow tumors but the medicine they had given her to shrink the tumors caused her liver to fail. The lung recipient has battled cystic fibrosis since birth and the heart recipient had a congenital heart defect. Once the teams had things dissected down to the aorta and vena cava the heart surgeon said he was ready for the heparin, which is a very strong blood thinner given in a dose that you would not give to someone who is alive. Anesthesia knew better than to give the heparin without talking to the TC and once it was confirmed that everyone was ready and each team had contacted their individual recipient teams, anesthesia gave the heparin. After five minutes the aorta and vena cava were clamped, we called it cross clamping, and that time was communicated over and over. It was the time the donor's heart stopped and the time when the clock started ticking down for the organs to be transplanted. The ice was dumped into the abdomen and chest. The silence of the monitor was so obvious in the OR at that point, it was abnormal to not hear it. There were many phone calls being made to communicate cross clamp. The heart always came out first, the surgeon lifted it out of the chest and walked to the back table with it in his hands. The lung team went to work in the chest as the heart surgeon inspected and flushed the heart. It was in perfect condition. He wrapped it in a lap sponge and held it against his body, thanked everyone and walked out of the room.

Two doors down to the right he would give someone a new life through another's death.

Things were happening so fast at that point there wasn't time to even think about the reality of the situation, which was probably good or you would be so overcome with emotion you wouldn't be able to do your job. It wasn't long before the lungs were out and the surgeons were so pleased with their condition they could barely contain their elation. The fact that these three recipients were all young women with so much life ahead of them fueled some of the emotions in the room. The liver team was starting as the lungs were flushed with cold preservation fluid, double bagged and packed in sterile ice inside a rolling cooler. Medical television shows love to show ridiculous scenes where the heart rolls out of a cooler that tips over in transport, which is totally impossible. Organs are double bagged and tied with zip ties, and both the bag and the outside of the box are labeled. The lung team came with our perfusionist, who couldn't leave until we were finished, so an ambulance was called to take them back and was ready and waiting for them to come down to the entrance so they could race them over to the recipient's hospital with their lights and sirens blaring. Every minute counts for lung and heart recipients, who are just about to the point of no return as the organ is in transport. Anesthesia was done and they cleaned up and left the room. The liver team kept working and the kidney team was assisting them. Sometimes the surgeon who recovers the liver also recovers the kidneys, but not this time. Their patient was critically ill and you could feel the tension in the team. The liver came out and, just like the rest of the organs, it was perfect. This young man took excellent care of his body and I silently thanked god that his young wife was brave enough to donate his organs, it would have been such a huge waste if she had not. Next, the kidney team worked. Once the kidneys were out the liver team usually stepped back in to get some extra blood vessels they would need to transplant the liver. The head liver surgeon was literally pacing alongside the table while the liver was being packaged.

There was no conversation except what was absolutely necessary. Every other sound seemed amplified because there was no beeping of the monitor. The liver surgeon had his resident call the recipient OR to check in and the news was not good, they were having trouble keeping her going and the decision was made to stop and wait for him to get back. He hung up and tore his gown and gloves off, announcing he was leaving without the vessels because if he didn't she would die. They were out the door and running down the hall to the helipad in seconds. We could only hope they would get back in time. The liver was backed up with other recipients if she didn't make it, so it wouldn't be wasted, but time would be against us if that happened. The kidney team finished up and my coworker scrubbed in to close the abdomen. We cleaned him up and the OR team brought in the morgue stretcher. We opened up the shroud kit on the stretcher, there were ties in the kit that you used to cross the patient's arms and tie them at the wrists. The other ties went around the ankles. The first toe tag is filled out and wrapped around the big toe, I grabbed his ankles and noticed the three rope bracelets were still there, then together we slid him over onto the bag and stretcher. I took the prayer card out of my pocket and placed it in his right hand where his wife had left it. I zipped up the bag, tied the other tag to the zipper and he was rolled out of the room.

I walked out into the hall to make a few phone calls, the first one to the medical examiner's office. I told the investigator that we were done and were ready for them to come pick the donor up, but there was one important detail I wanted them to know. I told him there was a prayer card in the donor's right hand that was placed there by his wife, and to please make sure it went back home with him. The next call was to the family. His brother answered the phone, I told him who I was and that we were finished. I told him the heart, lungs and liver were being transplanted into three young women, 24 and 25 years old. He said his family would be thrilled to hear that. I told him the pancreas and one kidney were going to a 50-year-old woman who would be cured of her diabetes and kidney failure by the transplant. Then I told him the other kidney was on it's way to the airport to be flown to their hometown, the brother didn't know at that point that their uncle was actually a match and was getting the second kidney.

I could hear his brother crying on the other end of the phone. He thanked me and I reminded him that they would get a letter from the TC who got consent in a couple weeks with more of the recipients' information (by then she would be able to find out how the recipients were doing post transplant). Five lives were saved that night.

As I packed my bags, I wondered how I was going to walk to my car because I was so tired. The circulating nurse came out of the OR where they were doing the heart transplant and motioned for me to come over. I walked over to the room and she said, "We are getting ready to come off bypass, want to watch?" I grabbed a new mask at the scrub sink and headed into the room. Anesthesia moved aside so I could stand up at the head of the table and the nurse grabbed me a standing stool. Across the OR table from the resident, the surgeon was standing with his arms folded, looking down at the heart inside the chest with his surgical loops and headlight. The heart monitor was silent and no one was talking. As the patient's blood started to flow directly into the heart I heard a single beep on the monitor, then another, then a few in a row, then a steady regular heartbeat. My brain was spinning trying to wrap itself around what I was witnessing. I could not control my emotions and I started to cry. I said to the surgeon that I couldn't believe it had started beating all by itself and he said, "It's a strong, healthy heart, it knows what to do." This was the only time in my two and a half years that I saw the heart literally give life to someone and I will never forget it. I left and drove home, very tired, mentally and physically, with many emotions beginning to surface. I made it home just about the time my daughters were leaving for school. I kissed them on their way out the door. My husband showed me the daily newspaper from the day before — it had a full-page picture of the boxer kneeling for his prayer before the fight in the ring. I looked at the picture and immediately my eyes went to his ankle. There were the three rope bracelets. The same ones that were on his ankle when I moved him into the body bag. All the feelings I had worked so hard to control all day and night came flooding out. I cried while I took a shower, I cried myself to sleep. From what I know all the recipients are doing extremely well.

■

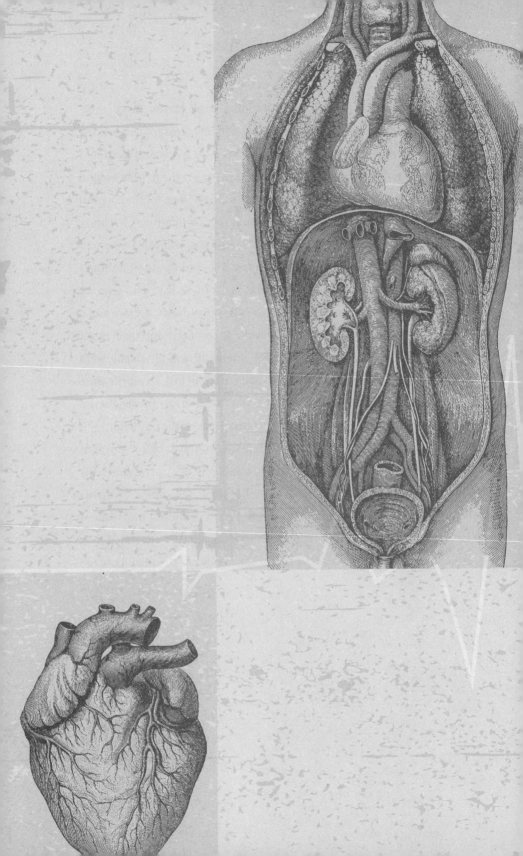

15

What I Have
Learned

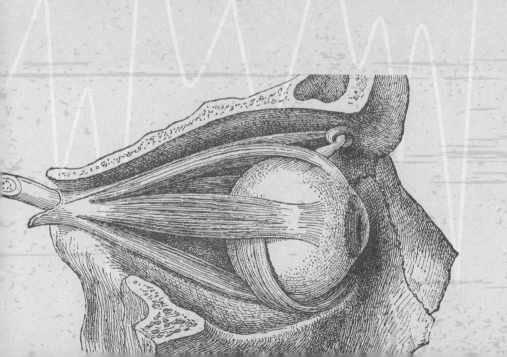

ICOULD NOT FINISH THIS BOOK WITHOUT WRITING ABOUT WHAT I HAVE learned personally from the experience of being an organ Transplant Coordinator. It was such a life-changing time that it really changed not only me but also many of the people around me who were impacted by my experiences. The daily interactions between myself, my husband and kids have been forever altered by this career. My husband and I never hang up the phone or say goodbye to our now 25-year-old son without saying "I love you." Our girls never leave the house without telling us they love us and us telling them the same thing. One day recently my youngest daughter left the house angry because we had had a fight about her choice of outfits. She slammed the door and did not respond when I yelled "I love you." When she came home later we had a very serious talk about what she would feel like if that was the last time she ever saw me, what if her last memory was of me yelling I love you and her ignoring it? It didn't take long before we were both bawling because we realized it was true, you never know what day will be your last. I'm 100 percent sure that, aside from a suicide, not one donor woke up the morning of their death and thought, I think I'm going to die today.

It seems everywhere I go somehow the topic of organ donation comes up and I am never quiet when it does. There are many strong opinions and beliefs among the public and the medical community. We are not organ vultures. We are not body snatchers. When I was speaking with a family who seemed to be hesitant about organ donation I would frequently explain that some people look at it as taking something from the donor, but we actually believed we were giving something to the donor, to the recipient and to the donor's family. We gave donors a chance to leave a legacy for their families, a way for them to literally save a life, even in their own death. Our organization never forgot any of the donor families. They were given grief-counseling services at our office and were made to feel a part of the donation family, that their contribution was recognized.

But, as I have said before, I try never to pass judgment on anyone in any circumstance. I think part of my reluctance to judge another person is my personality, part of it is how my life has gone and part of it is that I started my medical career in the Operating Room honestly. Here's what I mean by that, in the OR there are strict rules for maintaining sterility in everything you do. From the way you open a package to the way you hand something or unfold a drape, there is a process for everything with the goal of keeping it sterile. It is a black or white world, there are no gray areas, something is sterile or not, and if in doubt it's considered not sterile. You treat every single patient, no matter who they are, what brought them there, or what's in their past medical history the same way. We surgical techs didn't know very much about the patient in the OR but we knew what needed to be done and exactly how to help the surgeon. We literally did not have the information or ability to be judgmental of a patient. After spending 16 years in that environment, starting when I was only 19, those standards have become a huge part of who I am today.

When it comes to death, people can be judged at the worst time of their life and I don't think it's fair. Anyone who experiences a death will eventually need to deal with it internally. The grief counselor used to say there is only one way to deal with the grief of death and that is directly through it — you can't escape dealing with it. I have watched so many people reacting to tragedy in so many different ways and from so many socioeconomic classes that I have come to the conclusion that the people who handle loss the best are the people who have no regrets. Most of us in the medical field are well aware that death is an inevitable part of life, the great equalizer. Being an organ TC on the donor side took my mortality and shoved it in my face. It made me acutely aware that anything can happen at any time. I could allow that to terrify me, instead I choose to let it help me appreciate life and those lives around me. I believe that we all should "say what we need to say" as per John Mayer's song, "Even if your hands are shaking, and your faith is broken. Say it with you heart wide open." Live your life not being afraid to tell people how you feel. Be nicer to those around you, even if it's the homeless guy you walk past everyday as if he's invisible. I wish that all people would realize that every interaction you have with another person could potentially be your last or their last. There are no guarantees any of us will be here tomorrow. Many of us rush through our busy days never paying attention to the little things that matter until someone is taken from us suddenly. Did they know how I felt about them? Did they know how much I loved them? Do they know how sorry I am I didn't say it more? Do they know how much I will miss them?

When tragedy strikes and it is your turn to die it doesn't matter who you are or how old you are or how rich you are or how important you are. It really only matters at that point what kind of legacy you have chosen to leave on this earth.

■

Appendix:
Transplant Coordinator Checklist

Date of case:

Referral:

- Huddle with RN (Registered Nurse)/resident/attending
- Review hospital chart
- Start AOPO (this was what we called our own chart)
- Patient demographics/DD (donor designation)
- Review HPI/PMH/PSH (history of present illness/past medical history/past surgical history)
- Labs/CT scans/tests
- Height/weight
- ABO confirmation/T & S request (confirmation of blood type)
- Blood product administration
- Request full set labs
- Review plan with RN i.e., FBP (follow by phone)

Serologies/ Human Leukocyte Antigen (HLA): The time in the process that blood is tested for communicable diseases

- AOC (Administrator on Call) approval
- Qualified Specimen (meaning it is all of the donor's blood, no blood bank blood)
- Hemodilution sheet (algorithm that determines if a specimen is qualified based on patient's weight)
- Contact Labs Inc./Quick (outside lab and courier)
- OPO (Organ Procurement Organization) labels in appropriate places

Family Communication:

- Identification of LNOK (legal next of kin)
- Review of Consent/Disclosure form with NOK (next of kin)
- Identification of specific organs/tissues authorized
- Clarification of use of donation, i.e., transplant/research

- Description of recovery process
- Location of recovery
- Impact on burial plans/restrictions
- Family expense concerns
- Explanation of suitability evaluation
- Explanation of need for med/soc (20-page medical-social questionnaire)
- Disclosure regarding images during recovery
- Description of medical examiner involvement
- Funeral home arrangements
- Opportunity to ask questions
- Original consent form in hospital chart
- Consent/Disclosure form signed by hospital witness
- Medical examiner/Coroner clearance
- Physical assessment
- Med/soc (medical-social) assessment

AOC Communication: These were the times when it was mandatory that you call the administrator who was on call with you

- En route to hospital
- Initial evaluation to include:
- Admittance date/HPI/DT/CPR/PMH/PSH (DT is down time, or how long a patient was down without medical help; the AOC wanted to know if the donor required CPR and if so, how long)
- Neurological status including plans for pronouncement (what reflexes the patient has left)
- Hemodynamics/pressors (pressors are medications that support the blood pressure)
- LNOK/code status (legal next of kin and if the patient is a full code or full support)
- Pre-family communication/consent
- Pronouncement (brain death pronouncement)
- Medical examiner clearance
- Review of med/soc (medical-social)
- Clarification of plan moving forward
- Post echo/bronchoscopy/lung management results (echo is an ultrasound of the heart, bronchoscopy is a test that uses a scope to look inside the lungs)
- Pre-allocation/review of lists
- Confirmation of call teams/setting OR (operating room) time
- Review of allocation results
- Review of travel arrangements for teams
- During organ recovery PRN
- Cross clamp
- Anatomical abnormalities

- Pathology results
- Review of organ anatomy
- Changes in allocation
- Final review of distribution
- Wrap up case, post-case calls
- Before leaving hospital

APC Communication: These were the most appropriate times to speak with an Advanced Practice Coordinator for guidance

- Pre-AOC referral review
- Pre-family communication/consent
- Plan post-pronouncement/OPO standing orders
- Pre-AOC organ-specific review call
- Pre-AOC allocation call
- Full review one hour before set OR time
- Post-case/pre-AOC wrap up call

General donor management: These are all ranges of test results we liked to stay within

- Quantitative HCG for females > 10 (HCG is a test done for a hormone that indicates either pregnancy or a cancer)
- Ensure pronouncement documented
- SBP > 100-110/HR 60-140 (range we liked the systolic blood pressure and heart rate within)
- UOP 1-3 cc/kg/hr, 100 cc/hr (urine output range)
- CVP 2-6 (central IV line in the neck or chest that measures pressure within the heart)
- SpO2 > 95%, PaO2 80-100, pH 7.35-7.45, pCO2 35-45 (oxygen saturation and arterial blood gas ranges)
- Electrolytes WNL (sodium and potassium within normal limits)
- Glucose 80-250
- Hgb > 10/Hct > 30 (Hemoglobin and hematocrit desired range)
- Temp 36°C-37.5°C
- Ancef 1 g every 8 hours (an antibiotic we gave)
- Type and cross 4 units PRBC's (packed red blood cells, 4 units needed to be ready in case the donor needed blood in the OR)
- ABO with A subtyping (blood typing)
- Continuous cardiac/SpO2 monitoring (cardiac and oxygen monitoring)
- Central line access with CVP monitoring
- Continuous arterial pressure monitoring (preferably in left radial artery for arterial blood gases and BP [blood pressure] monitoring)
- Additional peripheral access X 2 (additional IV access sites)
- NG/OG tube (nasogastric/orogastric tube to drain stomach contents)

- Continuous documentation
- T4 protocol initiated (the levothyroxine IV we started)
- CXR (chest X-ray)
- Labs every 4-6 hours (Blood tests to monitor kidney and liver function every 4-6 hours)
- Blood/urine/sputum cultures (tests to ensure there are no infections)
- Tissue packs drawn, labeled and OTD (tissue packs are boxes with tubes of blood for kidney matching that would be labeled and couriered to interested hospitals, OTD means out the door)
- UA with micro (urinalysis with micro, looking for infection)

Organ-specific management: these were things we did to evaluate each organ individually

Heart:
- Echo/TEE within 12 hours of offer (post herniation) (Echo is an ultrasound of the heart)
- Copy of echo on CD (this goes with the heart team)
- Correct electrolytes (sodium and potassium need to be as normal as possible to keep heart functioning)
- Wean off pressors pre-echo if possible (we needed to get off as many blood pressure supporting medications as possible to get an accurate result)
- Possible dobutamine challenge with EF (Ejection Fraction) < 50 percent (if first echo gives result of EF < 50 percent we would run a drug that stimulates the heart like a stress test; EF is a calculation for how efficiently the heart is pumping, it does not mean the heart is working at 50 percent)
- EKG within 12 hours of offer, must be read
- CPK/troponins (cardiac enzymes that would indicate a heart attack/MI)
- Cardiac catheterization required on all males > 40, females > 45 (ensures there are no arterial blockages in the heart, is done on younger patients if there are significant risk factors like smoking)
- CXR (chest X-ray)
- ABG (arterial blood gas) within 3 hours of offer
- Strict I and O's (intake and output, measuring to be sure the donor is getting enough fluids)

Lungs:
- CXR within 3 hours of offer (chest X-ray)
- CXR every 8 hours with recent copies for team
- HOB up, pulmonary toileting every 2 hours (Head of bed up, pulmonary toileting is the term used for doing some light patting on the patient's back and/or chest to loosen any phlegm or fluid in the chest followed by suctioning)
- Albuterol puffs every 4 hours (inhaler used by asthmatics given through endotracheal tube)

- Hyperinflate ETT cuff (endotracheal tube or breathing tube, we hyperinflated the cuff inside to ensure we had no air leaks)
- Calculate tidal volume per 10-12 ml/kg for ideal body weight (calculation to determine the volume of the lung to ensure proper ventilation)
- ABG's every 4 hours, 30 min post vent change and change in pulmonary function (arterial blood gases done every 4 hours or if we made a change on the ventilator)
- Maintain Hgb > 10, HCT > 30, CVP 2-6 (Hemoglobin, hematocrit, CVP monitoring are all measuring blood volume)
- Solumedrol 1 g every 6 hours or 15-30 mg/kg (steroid given to help inflammation of the lungs and improve lung function)
- Serial ABG's every 6 hours (arterial blood gases)
- Maintain FiO2 80-100 on lowest FiO2 percent (setting on the ventilator)
- O2 challenge every 3-4 hours (this was like an exercise for the lungs that took about a half hour to complete, basically blowing them out to max capacity and holding it for a period of time)
- Sputum gram stain within 24 hours of offer (ensures no active infection in the lungs)
- Bronchoscopy (test to look inside the lungs with a flexible scope)
- Possible CT (cat scan)
- Review of ventilator settings (ensuring everything is set where it is supposed to be)

Liver:
- Trauma/prolonged DT (down time can affect liver enzyme tests)
- Obesity/BMI (Body Mass Index)
- Hepatitis
- ETOH/drug abuse (alcohol)
- LFT's, coagulates, NA, ABG's (blood tests that are affected by the liver function)

Kidneys:
- HTN/DM/UTI's, stones (hypertension, diabetes mellitus, urinary tract infections or kidney stones)
- BUN/creat, admit, trends (blood tests to level and track kidney function)
- Electrolyte disturbances (sodium and potassium)
- UA with micro at admittance, initiation of management, prior to OR (urinalysis to ensure no bacteria)
- Foley with urimeter (a special urine bag that measures urine output)

Pancreas:
- Amylase/Lipase/Glucose (blood tests to measure pancreas function)
- Insulin usage (did the donor use insulin before admission or during)
- Obesity/Diabetes Mellitus/Surgery/ETOH use (alcohol use)

Allocation: assignment of the organs to a recipient

- Review of donor profile on UNOS/donornet (computer program used nationwide for communication among donor organizations and transplant surgeons)
- Review and sign UNOS match run lists (lists with matching blood types for lungs, heart, and liver faxed to TC onsite, list of recipients in the order they are "listed")
- Discuss with AOC organs being allocated/suitability
- Identification of recipients locally
- Identification of recipients regionally
- Identification of recipients nationally
- APC/AOC review of allocation completion (doing a run down of what organs were placed for transplant plus their backups)
- Setting of OR time (coordinated with OR and anesthesia staff)
- Perfusion notified
- Transportation arrangements for teams
- Kidney on-call team notified if applicable
- Pathologist notified if applicable (hospital pathologists had to come in and do kidney biopsies and liver biopsies sometimes during the recovery in the OR)
- In-house transplant team offered to recover (only if you are at a transplant center)
- Confirmation of OR time/review of guidelines with OR charge nurse
- Confirmation of OR time/review of guidelines with anesthesia staff

1 hr prior to OR: list of things to be completed before heading to the OR

- Give 1 g solumedrol (peds 30 mg/kg) (steroid for the lungs)
- Give 1 g Ancef if > 4 hours since last dose (antibiotics)
- Increase FiO2 to 100 percent (percent of oxygen donor is getting from ventilator)
- Discontinue all anti-diuretics, vasopressin (stop any meds that were used to eliminate excess fluids or stop the donor from urinating too much, which happens sometimes with brain death)
- Review, update and fax record to OPO office donor
- Make chart copies for organ teams
- Pancreas cocktail ordered (a mixture of meds and Betadine we would insert into the nasogastric tube that sterilized the inside of the pancreas if it was being transplanted)
- Draw blood for BUN (Blood Urea Nitrogen)/creatine/electrolytes (lab tests for kidney function)
- Collect specimens for OPO cultures (another way of ensuring the donor has no active infections)
- Arrange for transport to the OR (transporting the donor is a process that takes multiple people)

- Portable life pack, 02 bag, valve, mask with a PEP valve (items necessary during transport to OR)
- Advanced Cardiac Life Support drug box
- Documentation in progress note of transport process

Intra-op donor management

- Introduce staff to recovery teams
- Confirm credentials and document
- Review necessary paperwork with surgeons
- Secure surgeon signatures
- Ensure 2 bovies/suctions (electrocautery used in surgery)
- Flash balfour (large abdominal retractor)
- Review drugs and timing with anesthesia staff
- Lasix 100 mg around time of incision (medication given to get rid of excess fluids)
- Mannitol 50 g around incision (medication given to pull excess fluid out of the liver)
- Muscle relaxant pre-incision
- Heparin 300 u/kg 5 minutes before cross clamp (blood thinner)
- Peds, 4 mg/kg lasix, 1 mg/kg mannitol (pediatric doses)
- Documentation and communication of cross clamp (multiple calls made at cross clamp)
- Blood tubes for perfusion
- Organ anatomy communicated to AOC
- Kidney anatomy communicated to AOC/OPO
- Biopsy results reported to AOC
- Appropriate specimens for tissue packs
- Review and sign all organs packaged for transport
- Review and sign organ distribution sheet
- Ensure operation notes signed and in hospital chart
- Postmortem care (the process of wrapping the hands and feet to be placed in the shroud or body bag)
- Postrecovery call to funeral home/medical examiner
- Medical examiner kit if requested (blood tubes drawn before heparin for medical examiner)
- Post-recovery call to family
- Wrap-up call to AOC
- Taped report call to OPO office for documentation purposes
- Hospital services coordinator emailed with outcome for follow up

Index